HALDOL AND THE HOLY SPIRIT

Also by Chet Caskey

100 Historic American Flags (2011)
Spokane's Historic Cemeteries (2012)
From Hats to Headbands (2013)
Let Us Never Forget That Our Enemies Are Men (2013)
The Amazing Strahorns (2013)
Haunted Spokane (2013)
Spooky Spokane (2015)
Confessions of a Religious Fanatic (2017)
Haunted Hillyard (2018)
Spokane Bedtime Stories (2019)

Haldol
and
The Holy Spirit

The thin line between devotion and madness

A Novel

by

Chet Caskey

Inland Cascadia Publications • Spokane • Washington

Haldol and The Holy Spirit: The thin line between devotion and madness
Copyright © 2021 Chester John Caskey & Catherine Ann Caskey

All rights reserved. No part of this publication may be reproduced, stored in a retrieval system, or transmitted in any form or by any means, electronic, mechanical, photocopying, recording, scanning, or otherwise, except as permitted under Section 107 or 108 of the 1976 United States Copyright Act, without the prior written permission of the publisher.

This is a work of fiction. Names, characters, places, and incidents are the product of the author's imagination or are used fictitiously. Any resemblance to real persons, places, establishments, or locales is entirely coincidental.

Book design: Gray Dog Press, Spokane, WA

Published by
Inland Cascadia Publications
818 West 29th Avenue
Spokane Washington 99203

ISBN: 978-0-578-96933-6

Printed in the United States of America

Acknowledgment

Special appreciation goes out to my life-partner and editor Catherine Caskey, without whose tireless assistance, multiple readings, and countless suggestions this book would have been considerably less readable than it is.

Madisonville, Iowa

1986

Haldol is the brand name of Haloperidol, the antipsychotic drug $C_{21}H_{23}ClFNO_2$ affecting the central nervous system and used in the treatment of Schizophrenia, Tourette Syndrome, Mania, Bipolar Disorder, Delirium, Agitation, Acute Psychosis and Hallucinations. Serious side effects, such as the movement disorder known as Tardive Dyskinesia, may occur with its use.

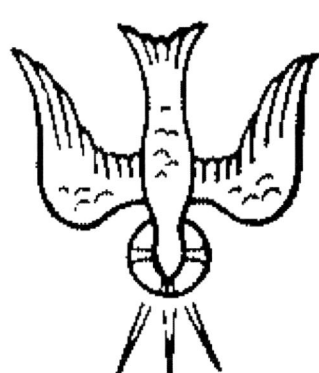

The Holy Spirit, in the Abrahamic Religions, is either an aspect or agent of God by means of which the Deity communicates with humans or interacts with them, often depicted as a descending dove.

Chapter One

"Tom," Sueann Schmidt said not looking up from her crocheting, "I think we need to get the boys christened or baptized or something."

"Baptized?" her husband Tom replied in exaggerated amazement. "We're not religious," he said. "We haven't been in a church since Tina and her deadbeat husband's wedding three years ago. Why don't we let the boys grow up and just decide for themselves if they want to be baptized – or not."

The whole idea of baptism and Christian rites gave Tom a bit of the creeps, but he had come by his aversion to religion rather honestly through both hearing of the experiences of his parents as young adults and listening to anecdotal stories from his older brothers growing up. Nevertheless, it was certainly not through a systematic consideration of the topic of religion that he had developed his spiritual allergy, despite a PhD in History and several compulsory papers he had written in college concerning the history and philosophy of religion.

His father Thomas Schmidt, Sr. had been raised in Cedar Rapids in a strict Roman Catholic family, and his father's sister had become a nun when she was sixteen. The elder Schmidt had been a product of Catholic elementary and high schools and had been an active Catholic even upon graduation from high school when he worked at Zoller Brewery. But then – at age twenty-four – he had attempted to get an annulment through the Church following a civil divorce in his first, and very brief, marriage to a woman considerably older than himself. After a short interview, his request for an annulment was flatly refused, and to add insult to his proverbial injury in a one paragraph ruling on the application from the Bishop of the Dubuque Diocese, he had been warned that re-marriage to anyone other than his former wife or as a widower would "imperil the immortal soul" within him.

Defiant or perhaps indifferent at that point, Tom Senior had remarried a Protestant three years later before a Justice of the Peace, only to receive a second one paragraph letter from the Bishop a week after he had confessed the details of the new union to his sister in the Mother of God Convent. This time the note related that his immortal soul was now in "the gravest of jeopardy" to the point that he was no longer authorized to take communion at mass. That ended Tom Senior's entire consideration of the Roman Catholic Church, and indeed all Churches, except for very occasional bitter railings and even fewer occasional fond reminiscences while in his cups with other Catholics.

Tom's mother Myrtle had been initially raised in the Fire Baptized Holiness Church in rural Hatch County in the northwest part of the State. In the 1920's the protestant churches of the Midwest were troubled and rocked by the pentecostal revolution, or "latter rain" revival, which had begun at the Azusa Street Baptist Church in Los Angeles in 1906. Congregations of Methodists, Presbyterians, and Nazarenes all over the country argued concerning the precise nature of the Holy Spirit, split with their brethren over tiny doctrinal differences, and split again.

In the East and Midwest several congregations of the fairly subdued Holiness Church became "pentecostalized" as the re-named Fire Baptized Holiness Church, and it was to one of these tiny groups that Myrtle's stern father Elmer led his family after leaving the Dry Creek Free Will Methodist Church. On Sunday mornings, and then on Sunday nights, and then again on Wednesday nights, the little congregation would sing, raise up holy hands, shout and extol the Holy Spirit to the point of dancing the Charleston in the aisles or lying in the pews clutching personal prayer cloths and weeping after becoming overcome with emotion.

However, it was not over the issue of the Holy Spirit that Elmer Howard left the Fire Baptized Holiness Church in 1934 with a contingent of three of the twelve families constituting the entire congregation. Rather, the bone of contention had been whether the New Testament supported the idea of preparing and serving communal meals and picnics on Church premises. Elmer had been a leader of the strict constructionist faction finding no such evidence in the Bible to support preparation of the meals and potluck dinners on church grounds that the larger group wanted to have. However, worshiping in the family's basement proved to be a poor substitute for the fellowship within an actual church building, and Elmer Howard died a troubled and bitter man at the age of sixty. Twelve years later, Myrtle's mother – on her own death bed – had told Myrtle she had seen "the devil in your father's eyes" the day he had told her the Lord Jesus was commanding the family to leave the Methodist Church in Dry Creek.

Perhaps not inexplicably as an adult and a mother, Myrtle herself displayed a highly skeptical and circumspect view of *all* religions, and in this respect she and her husband Tom Senior saw eye-to-eye on one of the few areas they were in agreement during their entire thirty-three-year marriage. They raised their three sons virtually devoid of all religious discussions, devoid of Sunday schools, and devoid of vacation bible schools save for the one summer when all three boys were shipped off to Hatch County to stay for six weeks with Myrtle's sister Hazel while Hazel's husband Galen nursed a broken leg and needed help with chores on the farm.

Farm chores under the critical eye of their crutch-bound, vile-mouthed and tobacco-chewing Uncle Galen would have been bad enough. However, whenever they were granted a respite from their seemingly endless chores that summer, they had to contend with their Aunt Hazel's self-appointed personal crusade to save their souls and atone for her atheistic sister's neglect of their religious education.

To get to their Aunt and Uncle's church, the boys rode in the back of their Uncle Galen's pick-up truck along the black top highway in front of the farm east for ten miles until they left the black top road for a gravel secondary road. Three miles later they left the gravel secondary road for a dirt tertiary road, and a mile and a half of dusty minutes down the dirt road they arrived at the white, one room little church house with a small slightly skewed steeple that had been tacked on to the peak of the roof as an ornamental afterthought.

The attendees of the church wore their very best to services, which meant for some of the men and boys bib overalls over a white shirt buttoned up at the collar without a tie. Because of lack of facilities everyone in the church, from toddler to centenarian, broke into age groups and huddled in this corner or that corner of the room for Sunday School, and then when Sunday School was over everyone re-assembled in the center of the church in the pews for the main service. The boys sat in the very back row of the room on the right-hand side, with the several other older boys. Two "elders", or senior men of the Church, stood by the door at the back in order to maintain needed order, particularly among the teen-age boys. Up front there was a piano played by one of the Sunday School teachers who was also the hymn leader for the congregation.

The preacher, one Gerald Mill, was not a graduate of any seminary and in fact not too many years earlier had been a diesel mechanic in Des Moines – and an active alcoholic. However, he wasn't an alcoholic without hope, and one day, as his own story in one sermon that summer went, he looked up "from the gutter and saw a vision of the Lord Jesus." He got off the hooch, procured a Bible, and became a self-ordained man of the cloth. He had heard the call to the ministry, and the Dry Creek Christian Church had taken him in to minister to them.

Preacher Mill was by all appearances a frustrated evangelist. His passion in the ministry was to "convert" the heathen, which was a most difficult task in a congregation consisting of forty people – all of whom over the age of ten had been baptized years, if not decades, before. This was a most unfortunate tendency of the preacher as it concerned the Schmidt brothers, because all through the summer of 1963 Reverend Mill set his sights on the conversion of the three young unsaved men to Christianity.

"Whosoever therefore shall confess me before men, him will I confess also before my Father which is in heaven", Reverend Mill would say quoting Jesus in the Book of Matthew, and he would add *"but whosoever shall deny me before men, him will I also deny before my Father which is in heaven – thus saith the Lord God, Beloved!"* After this, he would instruct Miss Melissa, the Sunday School teacher-pianist, to play the hymn *"Just As I Am"* as the congregation sang all four tortured verses of the song waiting for a sinner in general – and the Schmidt brothers in particular – to move to the center aisle and walk to the front.

When Reverend Mill became frustrated week after week that summer, he began to have Miss Melissa play the entire hymn three or four times interposed with exhortations, mini-sermons, lectures and even pleas to the tiny congregation pointing out that *surely* someone sitting somewhere in the congregation needed to come forward and be saved – even if only to repent of having "back slid" after they were saved the first or second time. But no one came forward, the Schmidt boys remained silent with their eyes frozen on the page of the hymnal containing the "*Just as I Am*" verses, and each service would end on a disappointed or frustrated note in Reverend Mill's voice.

As the end of the boys' summer in Hatch County began to draw to an end, their Aunt Hazel announced that arrangements had been made for Tom, Jr. – the youngest brother – to go to Christian Boys Camp in neighboring Smith County for an entire week of fun, games, and activities. This sounded appealing to Tom who envisioned a welcome escape from barn painting. However, upon arrival at the camp he discovered that the point of the camp was nearly exclusively the religious conversion of the ten- and eleven-year-old boys in attendance. During the day they had talks with counselors about Jesus, and at night – every night – they all attended a juvenile-oriented revival service. Each night three or four of the boys would emotionally break, rise from their metal folding chairs, and walk or run down the aisle of the meeting tent to say the Sinner's Prayer with the camp preacher, Brother Scott. Then, immediately and without parents or family members being notified or in attendance, the entire congregation of boys, camp counselors and Brother Scott would proceed over to the swimming pool singing "*Onward Christian Soldiers*", and the newly repentant boys would be baptized in the pool's shallow-end with Brother Scott standing waist deep in the water and dipping each boy backward "in the name of the Father, and of the Son, and of the Holy Ghost." To his Aunt Hazel's disgust, Tom returned to the farm "unsaved."

As dating young adults, Sueann had seemed to Tom, Jr. to be indifferent to religion, and outside of their own wedding ceremony at the Abundant Love Lutheran Church in 1977 and three other weddings of friends they attended in the succeeding years, the couple had not entered a church building together in their entire relationship. Sueann's parents had been life-long attendees, first at Good Shepherd Lutheran Church and then at the newly formed Abundant Love Lutheran Church when the larger congregation had decided to fund a new daughter-church in South Madisonville in 1968 as the city's suburbs grew across the Little Otoe

River. Sueann's parents had vociferously opposed any wedding except a traditional one and in the bride's own church. The church being affiliated with the Missouri Synod of the Lutheran Church, however, meant that Tom and Sueann were required to attend three "Pre-marital Counseling Sessions" prior to the wedding where the church's pastor and prospective officiate asked them questions like "have the two of you prayed together over the Christian goals for your marriage?"

During the last session of pre-marital counseling, the pastor had handed Tom a little hard-bound book entitled "*The Role of Physical Intimacy in Christ's Plan for Marriage*," as he said "folks, we have to face the fact that sex is a part of marriage." Sueann had burst out laughing at the remark – and despite it becoming more and more embarrassing as the thirty-minute session ground to an end – she continued to periodically laugh into her hand to the point of having to excuse herself from the room. The couple had already been living together for three years, and Sueann was nearly three months pregnant – a fact that officially had escaped her father's attention but which fully justified a February wedding as far as her mother was concerned. For years Tom had kept the book on the shelf between Miller's "*History of the Dark Ages*" and a novel entitled "*A Marriage of Convenience*" as a private joke between Sueann and him – but Sueann didn't seem like she was less than serious now.

"Did you hear me?" Tom asked after a few seconds of non-response form Sueann.

"Yeah, I heard you," Sueann answered. "It just seems to me," she continued, "that from a perspective of family life it's something *we ought to do*. Linda and I were both baptized as babies by Mom and Dad at Good Shepherd. Timmy is already four years old, and the baby's still an infant. Let's baptize them both now and just get this aspect of family life over with."

"You've been listening to Shirley, I take it?" Tom said sarcastically.

"No, I have not been *listening* to my mother!" Sueann retorted. She hated Tom's condescending references to her mother and the demeaning choice of words he always used as if her mother were issuing her instructions rather than simply having a conversation with a grown daughter and the mother of two. In fact, she *had* talked about the baptismal issue with

Shirley, but it was out of the question that she could ever admit to even such an insignificant thing without Tom making a big deal out of it and implying she didn't have a mind of her own. Besides, Tom didn't want her to have a mind of her own, she thought. What he wanted was for her to have *his* mind as *her* own.

"These boys are eventually going to want to go to college," Sueann continued, "and that college just might be Harvest Christian University right here in Madisonville or Exeter Lutheran over in Hildreth. Or, they just might want to get a decent job one day and support themselves and be interviewing with a Christian boss who wonders why he should hire an unchurched kid who was raised by a couple of atheists. It's like smoking, Tom. Nobody is going to complain that you *don't* smoke at your desk and annoy co-workers. It's the smokers who have to worry these days about irritating someone, and that someone could be their boss. We live in a Christian country, and it's not the Christians who have to worry about raising eyebrows at work or losing out on the chance of getting nice Christian girlfriends because it comes out in conversation on the first date they are heathens."

"I don't know," replied Tom. "It came out that I was a heathen on our first or second date, and I still ended up with a nice Lutheran girl."

"Tom, I mean it. I'm serious," Sueann said. "If you want to be the rebellious intellectual history teacher at Harvest Christian and wear your atheism proudly on your sleeve, then do it. But don't penalize our boys."

"I am not an atheist!" Tom replied indignantly. "Privately I am a very spiritual person – just non-conforming in traditional faiths."

"Look," continued Sueann, "you've been a special lecturer in European History for five years. They made Mike Boston an Associate Professor two years ago. I know you're not in the Math Department, but how about 2 + 2 equaling no Associate Professorship for an atheist at a Christian university?"

"For crying out loud!" said Tom getting up. "Go ahead and baptize the boys! Pick a church! I'll come in a coat and tie and praise the Lord with you."

"Not good enough," replied Sueann in a calm voice as she continued crocheting. "This is a family thing. I want you to be part of the process.

You are the boys' father – the patriarch of our family in Judeo-Christian terms. I want you to pick the church with me."

"That'll be the day," Tom muttered as he walked into the kitchen for a beer. "Jesus H. Christ."

Chapter Two

Still, Sueann's remarks about the professional practicality of being a Christian began to trouble Tom. PhDs in the Liberal Arts were a proverbial "dime a dozen" these days, and job placement for college level teachers was tough – especially in the Midwest where curricula were changing toward an emphasis on business and technical sciences and away from the humanities as legitimate undergraduate degrees. Just this academic year the University had done away with the foreign language requirement for all but a handful of majors, and next year one of the history survey classes he taught freshmen would become interchangeable with a survey class in political science, art history or philosophy in order to fulfill the humanities requirement for an undergraduate degree. One didn't need a PhD in history to know that historically when jobs became tight, those with greater seniority would force the relative newcomers out of their positions if push came to shove. In academia "survival of the fittest" meant achieving tenure *before* a crisis hit, and in order to obtain tenure he would have to advance to at least an Associate Professorship in the immediate future.

At a Faculty Senate meeting the next week in which his sub-committee was considering recommendation of the proposed new student handbook, Tom happened to flip to the front page of the booklet as Professor Thompson from the School of Engineering was making some rambling point about the proposed honor system relative to plagiarism when his eyes fell upon a one paragraph pre-amble to the pamphlet. It read:

Mission Statement
It is the overriding and divinely favored purpose of Harvest Christian University to foster a distinctly New Testament atmosphere for morally committed students to complete their studies in higher education

within a Godly environment mentored by a highly qualified staff of like-minded teaching professionals."

"Well," thought Tom to himself disgustedly. "I have about as much chance of making tenure here as the devil himself." As Ms. Hildebrandt of the Art Department politely took issue with Professor Thompson's last remarks, Tom thought that he only really had two viable options. The first was to update his resumé and start sending it out. Maybe Iowa State – but someone told him at the Faculty Club awhile back that Iowa State wasn't hiring in the College of Liberal Arts. It was always risky to send out resumés and not have it get back to the Department.

Then again, "maybe Sueann was on to something on the Christian thing," Tom thought. "Really, what would it hurt to play the game? After all, it couldn't be any more nauseating and hypocritical than the entire academic field was to begin with. He could rationalize being a Christian in his own mind along the lines of the basic scenario he was already committed to in order to support the family."

"What do you think about this issue of signed honor pledges, Mr. Schmidt?" the Committee Chairman suddenly asked invading Tom's focused preoccupation with his own thoughts. Tom didn't have a clue as to what discussion had ensued in the last few minutes.

"I think," Tom replied sagaciously, "that I would like to consider the point further – perhaps *even pray about it*. Isn't that what we are all about here, education-wise?"

"Point well taken, Tom," Professor Thompson said smiling.

That evening when Sueann stuck her head into the boy's bathroom to see how the baby's bath was progressing, Tom looked up from the floor by the tub with a Pooh Bear towel flung over his shoulder and one hand on Terry.

"Sueann," Tom said smiling. "I've been thinking that I might do you one better on this church thing we were talking about Sunday. Why don't we *all* join a church – you know, as a family. You were baptized as a child. I could get christened or baptized or whatever with the boys, and then all your men would be saved! Would that appeal to you?"

Sueann stood in the doorway slightly stunned. Instead of making a joke of it or even acknowledging Tom's wide smile and half-laugh, she simply said quietly, "Tom, I would like that very much. I know it doesn't mean a great deal to you, but it would mean a lot to me. Thank-you."

"Well then, it's settled," Tom said guarding his face with the palm of his outstretched free hand as Terry made sudden splashes with both hands in the tub. "I suggest we visit some churches over the next few weeks and see if one appeals to us – that is, of course, unless you would rather us just join Good Shepherd or Abundant Love Lutheran."

"No, no," Sueann replied turning her head to focus again on Tom and suddenly coming back into the conversation after staring for a moment off into space. "Not Lutheran. Let's start our own family tradition."

"Fine," said Tom smiling as he reached out his wet free hand to touch her knee.

In the ensuing weeks Tom tried very much *not* to think of himself as the hypocrite he clearly knew he was in his more introspective moments. His only comfort was in the thought that the Baby Jesus, Virgin Mary, and that Holy Ghost stuff was undoubtedly all a bunch of hogwash to begin with, so that his noble gesture in agreeing to Sueann's desire for a familial spirituality was – from the standpoint of relative ethics – probably a "good deed."

Then even that rationalization failed as Tom admitted to himself that Sueann had little or nothing to do with his hypocrisy. He wanted tenure. He wanted permanency. In a way maybe he even wanted a type of *respectability* from his peers he had never really felt before. However, without a doubt and even in the deepest depths of his rationalizations, personal salvation, rescue from Armageddon and things like that were irrelevant to his newfound religiosity.

After a completely miserable first Sunday at the First United Methodist Church on Fifth Street when the baby would not keep still and Timmy crawled under the pews and out of sight between rows of seated legs during the sermon, Sueann and Tom agreed that the first criterion for the new church – the *sine qua non* of church membership – would have to be whether or not the congregation had a nursery or "cry room" for both of the boys. The First United Methodist Church had not. The Presbyterian Church they called did not.

The Congregational Church did have a cry room, but when the New Members Committee made a house call on the family three days after the Schmidts attended a service and filled out a Visitor's Card the committee so annoyed both Sueann and Tom that the Congregational Church was x-ed off of their list of possibilities. The committee of three male "elders" rang the doorbell right at meal time when the boys were both being monstrous – and moreover they all stood in the foyer of the house for the better part of thirty minutes without grasping the most blatant of hints that they had come at the wrong time.

"Blasted Jehovah's Witnesses show more decency than these guys!" Tom exclaimed when he was finally able to shut the front door behind them. Sueann agreed.

However, on the third Sunday of their reconnaissance they seemingly had a stroke of luck. St. Albans Episcopal Church was an imposing building at the corner of Eighth Street and Maple surrounded by an ornate fence of freshly painted black iron. The 19th Century Gothic Revival structure of the church itself was almost a hundred years old, but the entire physical plant consisting additionally of an architecturally complementary large parish hall, church offices, an elementary school through grade three, and an extensive playground took up the entire block. The church was constructed of rough-hewn gray stone trimmed in white stone arched windows and doorways. The tall bell tower displayed four large clock faces on each side near the roofline, each with the correct time displayed, no less.

Neither Tom nor Sueann had ever been in an Episcopal Church, but they both liked the building enough to want to see the inside of it during a service. Sueann had heard that it was "like Catholic, only more liberal." In as much as Tom was in favor of any amount of liberalism in religion, however couched, upon discovering that the Church had a nursery during services the two agreed that St. Albans would be their next adventure.

When the St. Albans Sunday arrived, both Tom and Sueann were impressed with the Church. The lush carved red oak panels, richly upholstered pews, beautiful stained-glass windows, and mini-cathedral ceiling with arching oak beams were aesthetic ornaments they had not yet seen outside of their one summer in Europe when Tom was in graduate school. Moreover, the Church, which Tom subsequently learned was richly endowed in funds from generations of former members, could afford to hire a classical organist, gifted musical director and partially professional choir for the music portions of the service. This was as far from Miss Melissa and her piano at the Dry Creek Christian Church as Handel was from Blue Grass banjo music. The classical music and the choir soloists on the Sunday of the Schmidt's visit were outstanding.

Best of all, the Episcopal priest's sermon seemed both erudite and charming to Tom, and it was sprinkled with literary and historical references obviously geared to an educated university town congregation's taste. There was no alter call. The priest did not beseech sinners to repent, and indeed during the sermon Jesus Christ was not even referred to directly. The congregation was well dressed, and Tom recognized several faculty members from the university including the department heads in English, Drama, and his own History among the pews. Sueann filled out a Visitor Card from the little wooden hymnal rack in the pew and dropped it into the collection plate when it came around.

Instead of an unannounced knock on the door at suppertime during the following week, Sueann received a call at home from one of the Assistant Priests at St. Albans, a Father Ben Grey, who made an appointment to come by and chat one evening when it was convenient to both Tom and Sueann. The chat, when it came, was low key and social with Father Grey agreeing to sharing a glass of wine with the Schmidts when asked by Tom.

When questioned about their specific desires by the priest, Tom mentioned the baptism of the two boys, and then said, "I am thinking myself of becoming a member of St. Albans so that I can sponsor the boys along with Sueann at their christening, but I'm not baptized. Exactly how does that work – you don't have to get up in front of the congregation or make a confession of sins or anything like that do you?"

The fact that the department head was a member of St. Albans was almost too good to be true. However, Tom was already thinking that the flip side of the good news in having his department head as a fellow member of St. Albans would be the humiliating bad news of having to demonstrate publicly he was *becoming* a Christian as opposed to having already *been one* since infancy. Indeed, the danger of even inadvertently intimating he was being his hypocritical self in joining St. Albans in the first place by such a public display might be a deal killer with regard to his joining the congregation formally. If that was a danger, Tom thought, it would be better to simply accompany Sueann to church and *pretend* to be a longstanding Episcopalian than risk being thought a Johnny-come-lately or opportunist.

"Not to worry," Father Grey said, instantly grasping the point as if he read Tom's mind. "We have a special provision in cases such as this. We do *private* baptisms for adults in our chapel by appointment."

"You mean no alter calls, no Sinner's Prayer and no public baptism?" Tom asked.

"You can have that if you want," the priest said, "and we don't like to baptize babies privately – but we do. However, it's often preferable for adults to have a *private* ceremony."

Tom smiled broadly. He liked this church more and more, and it seemed to answer every problem posed in his exposure to Christianity growing up. At St. Albans he could be an aesthetic and culturally Christian hypocrite in an erudite and socially sophisticated traditional church without the emotional public passion, the calls on the name of the "Lord Jesus", or the anti-intellectual church services. Moreover, in terms of advancement of his career, he could think of no Christian denomination more traditional, more stable, or more dependable than the Episcopalian Church. Yes, he would become an Episcopalian, he thought. He actually looked forward to it.

The next day Tom called Father Grey, and he made an appointment for his private baptism in the St. Albans' Chapel the following week.

"How marvelous that God has spoken to you in such a dynamic way," the priest said on the phone.

On November 30, 1981 at 11:30 a.m., Tom met the Assistant Priest in the little chapel off to the side of the church office at St. Albans to be baptized. Sueann was the lone sponsor and witness other than the priest.

"Do you renounce Satan and all the spiritual forces of wickedness that rebel against God?" Father Grey asked Tom in the brief ceremony.

"Oh, yes," Tom answered, "I renounce *all* of them."

"Do you renounce the evil powers of this world which corrupt and destroy the creatures of God?"

"Yes," Tom said matter-of-factly.

"Do you renounce all sinful desires that draw you from the love of God?"

"I renounce them all," Tom replied.

With a silver cup, the priest dripped a few drops of water on Tom's head three times, immediately followed by dabbing the spot with a small monogrammed linen towel. Then juggling the towel and his prayer book, he announced, "I baptize you in the name of the Father and of the Son and of the Holy Spirit. Amen."

That was it. Tom was a Christian, at least formally. It hadn't seemed all that bad, actually. Tom shook Father Grey's hand and invited him to join Sueann and him for lunch at the Faculty Club. The priest politely declined and retreated back toward the church offices.

"I'll get the car, Honey," Sueann said squeezing Tom's hand. "Why don't you take a minute privately in here if you like and meet me outside by the Eighth Street entrance."

"Okay," Tom said submissively, although he didn't really see what Sueann was driving at. However, as soon as he was alone Tom inexplicably began to get emotional, and even wiped back the very beginning of a tear in the corner of his right eye. Tom had never prayed, not once, and not even when Reverend Mills had commanded that every head be bowed, and every eye be closed for prayer at the Dry Creek Christian Church that summer when he was ten. He had silently *not* prayed when his teachers had led the class in the Lord's Prayer after the Pledge of Allegiance in kindergarten and grade school. He had *not* prayed that the Cubans would not fire their missiles at the United States in sixth grade or that the Communists would not attack Madisonville with bombs and paratroopers. He had *not* even prayed that his Grandmother Howard not die when his mother had told him she was in fact dying. But now. But now, he felt a prayer forming in his mind as he stood silently in the chapel. It would do no good, of course. There was no God and even if there were, the deity was unlikely to be standing by to hear his prayer out of hundreds of millions of prayers uttered by really, truly sincere Christians. Still . . . Tom folded his hands and – moving in between two rows of pews, pulled down the kneeler and kneeled down upon it.

Looking up to the ceiling of the chapel, he began to say out loud, "God – if there is a God. If you are there and are not a total figment of mass hysterical imaginations, then show me yourself. Appear to me. Speak to me."

"If not . . ." Tom thought silently, "well, if not then there is nothing *up there* or *out there* or even *in here* except a fool. A hypocritical fool named Tom Schmidt." There was seemingly no point in going on, and Tom rose up and instinctively brushed off his trousers, but there was nothing to brush off. The little chapel's kneelers and even floor were as immaculate and spotless as everything else at St. Albans. He walked out of the chapel and through the Eighth Street entrance to meet Sueann.

Chapter Three

For two years Tom and Sueann threw themselves into church life at St. Albans. Sueann joined the Garden Guild and enjoyed working throughout the various seasons in the beautifully landscaped church grounds. First Timmy, and then Terry, were enrolled in St. Albans School. On special Sundays, the Schmidt parents would witness with pleasure little pageants and choral pieces put on by the school children as a part of the Sunday Family Eucharistic Service.

For his part, Tom accepted a nomination and appointment to the twelve-member Associate Vestry at St. Albans whose primary job was securing monetary pledges from church members residing in his assigned neighborhood. In the first year of his appointment, to his amazement one of the names on his contact list was Professor Emory, the head of the History Department at Harvest Christian University. On the appointed evening when Tom rang the professor's doorbell, he was greeted by his supervisor at the door with a broad smile and a warm handshake.

"Come in, come in Schmidt!" the professor said enthusiastically.

"Oh, this is for you," the professor said handing Tom an envelope. "It's our yearly pledge – been the same since 1976. But, come in! Let's sit down in the library over a glass of port and talk about history!"

They hadn't really talked about history that evening, of course. Professor Emory wanted to know all about Tom's primary areas of interest and what kind of scholarly works Tom had in progress.

"A comparative study, actually," Tom lied. "I am interested in how the Byzantine transformation to Orthodox Christianity beginning with the Emperor Constantine compares to the Roman Catholic Counter-Reformation a millennium later. Perhaps it will only be a manuscript. Perhaps a full-length book. It's not clear at this early stage, but the comparison between essentially state endorsed priesthoods in both instances on primitive Christianity initially and subsequently on neo-primitive Christianity in the Reformation is something that needs looking into."

"Fascinating!" the professor had said. "I hope you will keep me in the loop as your study progresses. You know, at some point in time as your career develops, you will need to regularly be putting these projects out into the academic world in print for all of us to share."

The evening had been encouraging beyond Tom's wildest expectations, and actually a thing not of his planning or manipulation at all. Professor Emory's name had just showed up on his contact list as if by – well, "as if by coincidence," Tom thought to himself as he endeavored to crowd out all thoughts of possible divine intervention.

While Professor Emory was replaced by Professor Hargrave as Department Head at the commencement of the next academic year, within six months following that, Tom was nevertheless elevated to an Associate Professor position at the university with a salary increase and a new graduate level course assignment: *The Comparative Development of Historical Trends in Christian Europe.*

"*See?*" Sueann said ecstatically when Tom had announced the good news.

"See what?" Tom asked ingenuously smiling.

"Oh you!" Sueann had responded with an exasperated tone of voice. "If you don't see God's hand in this then you aren't smart enough to be an Associate Professor."

Actually, Tom *had* vaguely and ever so tenuously begun to see God's hand in it, or so he thought. Things were happening in ever-increasing good measure in his life. His marriage with Sueann had never seemed happier. Sueann herself seemed happier. The boys were well adjusted in school, and the family could now afford a second car, and they put the idea that Sueann ought to get a job outside of the house finally behind them.

Then one Saturday Tom received a call from Father Earl Brickwood, the Pastor or head Priest of St. Albans, to request that he please come to his office when convenient. While Tom now was well acquainted with the Assistant Priest Father Grey and had even played golf with him once in a church tournament, Tom had never actually met the Pastor in charge personally before or seen his office.

As he entered his office's large oak (and open) door, Tom was impressed with the luscious oak paneling, walls of bookcases crowded with beautiful leather-bound books, and a fireplace centered on one wall large enough to walk into. Father Brickwood's office seemed like something out of a Nineteenth Century gothic novel. The meeting was brief and to the point. The priest had a small book he was giving Tom to read if Tom had time. The book was Henri Nouwen's *Prayer of the Heart*, and from the looks of the half-shelf full of copies Father Brickwood had on hand, Tom was not the only recipient of the recommended reading.

However, when he looked over the book later it seemed to be a strange offering from the priest, and certainly not any type of reading for a general audience. In fact, Tom could not fathom why the priest would have given even an academic such a book. The book dealt with a bizarre and esoteric topic Tom had only become familiar with through graduate studies concerning the Byzantine Empire: hesychastic prayer of Fourth and Fifth Century Christian monks and hermits in the Egyptian desert. These so-called "Desert Fathers" had developed a meditative system of continual dialogue with God through messages sent and *received* allegedly through the continual beat of their hearts, hence the popular name of the practice as "Prayer of the Heart."

Nevertheless, as strange as the book seemed, Tom became fascinated with it and found that he could not put the thing down that afternoon. It was two in the morning before he finished the book. On Monday he checked out the only two books concerning the Desert Fathers on the shelves at the university's library, and an hour later at the university's bookstore he ordered all six of the *Books in Print* pertaining to hesychastic prayer, the Desert Fathers, or Fifth and Sixth Century Monasticism. One of the books was in German. Tom read them all, and then he read them all again.

According to St. Gregory Palamas, Tom learned, hesychastic prayer produced a total physical and emotional ecstasy as the "Uncreated Light" of the Holy Spirit flooded into the human heart. The idea that the human heart could be a conduit to communication with God began – in small ways – to occupy more and more of Tom's thinking when he was alone. Didn't the Roman Catholics have this graphic image of the exposed heart of Jesus bound by a crown of thorns and a flame? "Maybe the Catholics as well as the ancient orthodox Christians were on to something," Tom thought to himself.

At some point in time and looking back, Tom could never determine just when that point in time had been, but Tom had ceased questioning in his own mind whether or not God existed. In fact, Tom now *knew* God existed. It was an old saying that a miracle is a coincidence seen through the eyes of faith. Before the point of balance in Tom's life, he had not believed in God. After that point, Tom ceased to believe in coincidences. There were simply too many unlikely life events now for them to be considered coincidences any longer. The great remaining question in Tom's mind had become the extent – if any – God communicated with humans. However, Tom already knew the answer to that question. They had done it. In the quiet and solitude of the Egyptian desert in the Fifth and Sixth Centuries – without traffic noises or television sets or electric mixers or cocktail party babble – they had *actually* done it. The monks had heard God speak to them *continually* through the beating of their own hearts. Continually. Without ceasing, like God was broadcasting through some radio signal.

Hadn't he heard a Bible verse long ago? Tom racked his memory. The Apostle Paul, "pray without ceasing." Yes, it all was beginning to make sense, Tom thought. God speaks to us continually and without ceasing. We just need to tap into that source – that heartbeat – and answer "yes, God, I am here. I am finally tuned in."

After Tom's discovery of the possibilities embraced through a meditative Prayer of the Heart he actually began to pray – and this time in earnest. To Sueann's utter amazement, he began to say a prayer at the commencement of the evening meals when they ate together as a family, and he began to make a point of tucking the boys into bed at night so that he could recite "Now I lay me down to sleep" with the children. Tom purchased his own copy of the *Episcopal Book of Common Prayer* in order to read and recite the recommended Daily prayers for each day of the year. He carried his prayer book in his briefcase to school in order to recite the daily prayers recommended for the noon hour, or "none" as the prayer was traditionally referred to. Eventually he began to suggest in earnest to a rather reluctant Sueann that the couple pray together as man and wife after the boys were put down for the evening.

"Aren't you carrying this prayer thing a bit far?" Sueann asked. "I mean I don't want to discourage you, and I'm delighted that you are so into St. Albans and the Christian family thing – but on the other hand it's just the two of us here. I mean if *you* want to pray feel free to. I'm just not comfortable in praying . . ."

"What?" asked Tom. "Praying with your husband? We've had two children together and have been lovers for over a decade. We presumably already pray together on Sunday in church. Why can't a man and a woman pray together in their own living room? What's more intimate – having sex or praying together?"

"I'm not sure," replied Sueann. "It's a new concept for me, really. Kind of creepy or scary in a way."

"You know, Sueann," Tom said, "either God answers prayer – or he doesn't. Isn't that sort of an axiomatic? If God doesn't answer prayer, then nothing is really lost in saying a little prayer together. But then again if God does answer prayer – what about those possibilities?"

"What do you want to pray for?" Sueann answered a bit sarcastically. "A new car?"

"No, no, no," Tom said. "That prosperity stuff is for holy rollers, and I'm not into that. How about praying – *for Timmy and Terry*? How about – '*Lord make our marriage strong in friendship and love for all time?*' "

"Oh, for heaven's sake!" said Sueann. "You make it difficult to turn you down. Get over here on the couch and I will pray with you. You do the lead praying. I'll do the assisting praying by silently agreeing with you. But we're not going to go on and on and get crazy, are we?"

"No, no, Sueann," Tom said. "Just a little prayer. Just a little meditation. Then a little silence in order to listen to our hearts. That's all."

Actually, Tom really wasn't all that interested in wordy prayers. Of the seven "species" of prayer defined in the back of the Episcopal prayer book the kind of prayer Tom was fascinated in was not mentioned. Prayer of the Heart. He wasn't exactly sure how Prayer of the Heart had worked for the Desert Fathers despite his reading, but he thought that if he could simply and frankly pray mechanically more and more – then the day would come when he could literally "pray without ceasing" through his beating heart and still carry on with his teaching, his conversations with others, and a whole host of daily activities. Then, he hoped, the "Uncreated Light" the Desert Fathers talked about might come streaming into his own heart and he would *hear God speak*. He would *feel God's presence*, and not just in some intellectual rationalized way he was sure even Father Brickwood was alluding to in some of his sermons. He would *experience God*. Hear God. Feel God. Ecstasy.

Tom had taken LSD twice in college and smoked enough marijuana in his twenties to make a bale. But that's not what he wanted. Tom didn't want intoxication. In fact, he seldom drank alcohol now – even at the Associate Vestry's wine and cheese parties. What he wanted was the fully sober and truly mind-blowing *ecstasy* that could only come from interacting directly with God. He wanted to be like Moses and be so close to God that he risked incineration if he looked God directly in the eye.

"Jesus Christ!" Tom thought to himself at times, "If I didn't have Sueann and the boys to worry about I would hock everything I have, fly to Egypt and disappear into the desert myself." He hadn't wanted anything so desperately before in his life. He wanted to actually experience God with every part of his being.

Of course, Tom couldn't tell anyone any of this. "I have to play the game," he thought to himself. He couldn't tell Sueann things like this. She was happy with the Garden Guild at church and a few socials. She even acted like she really wasn't listening to the sermon on Sundays or getting anything out of the service. The men in the Associate Vestry were more interested in the latest California wine and a source for Cuban cigars. At the university . . . Well, at the university it was all well and good to *act like* a Christian. To play the game and go to church and shuffle up to the front alter rail for communion – but to actually be a *real* Christian? Not to pretend, but to pray for a purpose and long to experience God? "Well, there probably wasn't a handful of *real* Christians in the entire university," Tom thought, "and that went for Professor Hargrave as well. He was a big hypocrite, and really had no business being the head of a department at an ostensibly Christian university."

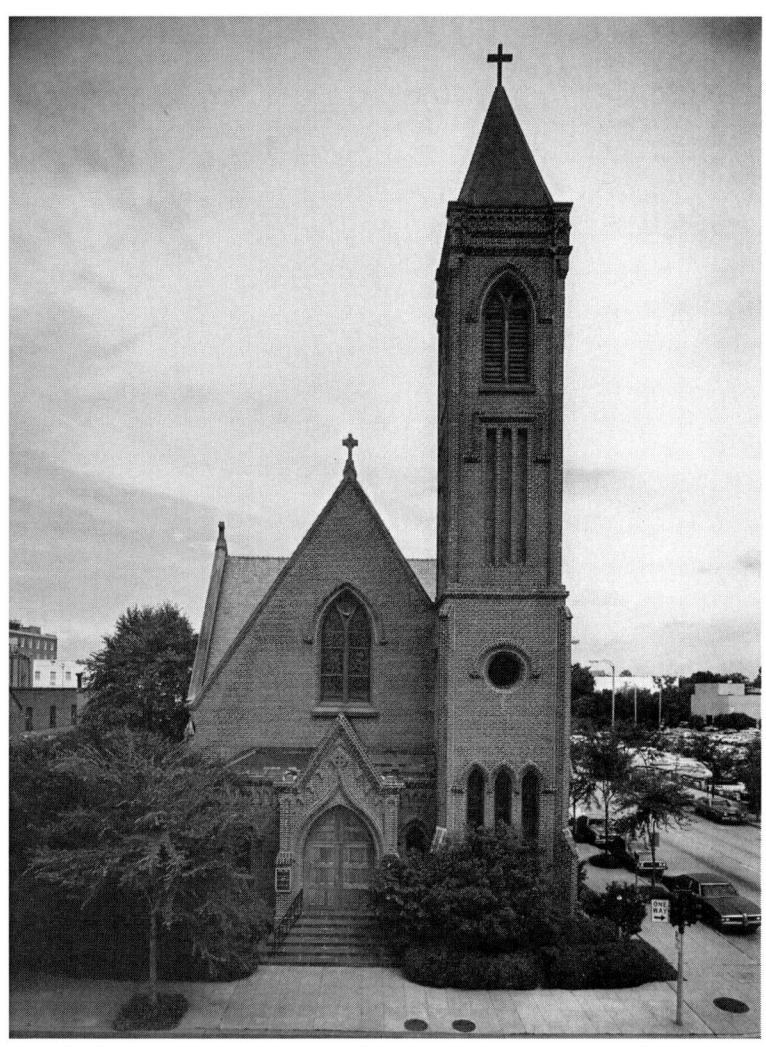

Chapter Four

Almost by accident Tom caught a glimpse of a flier thumb-tacked to the hallway bulletin board outside of the parish hall at St. St. Albans one late November Sunday in 1988 after the coffee hour, which was really only about fifteen minutes long and followed the 10:30 service. The bulletin announced:

ADVENT AWAKENING
December 5, 1988
7 p.m.
Hilton Hotel, Airport Drive, Madisonville
Join Episcopal Bishop David Blessing in an Evening of Renewal
Music by The Divine Lights

The "Advent Awaking" caught Tom's interest, but exactly why he could not then say. Certainly, *subsequently* he would have many theories as to why he became interested in going, and then changed his mind when Sueann refused to go with him, and then changed his mind again and decided to go by himself anyway.

The huge Ball Room at the Hilton Hotel had been subdivided with a large partition to create a more intimate enclosed space for the little conference. When Tom arrived, he found that even subdivided, the *ad hoc* meeting room was only half full of participants. As he walked into the function everyone was standing and singing. The Divine Lights Christian folk singers were standing on a little platform with three Spanish guitars and a female vocalist.

A young woman was leading the congregation of perhaps two hundred in a song, but the selection was neither traditionally classic like the music at St. Albans nor like the Salvation Army marching songs plinked out on the piano by Miss Melissa at the Dry Creek Christian Church. Song after song was sung in an unhurried way as Tom stood at the back of the room. There weren't any song sheets or hymnals provided for the group, but the songs – almost childlike in their simplicity – were so melodious and repetitious that everyone knew the words and the melodies by the second time through, and each verse was sung many times.

Lord, you are more precious than silver.
Lord, you are more costly than gold.
Lord, you are more beautiful than diamonds,
And nothing I desire compares to you.

Tom thought the simple songs were very peaceful, and nobody seemed in a hurry to get through the singing and "get on with" the program. Then Tom noticed that about half the crowd was lifting up one or both hands during the songs. Tom thought to himself that this exercise wasn't just singing hymns like he had experienced in church. These people were singing, but they were also engaged in a form of *worship* and *prayer*, which like Prayer of the Heart was not defined in the back of the *Episcopal Book of Common Prayer*. Moreover, Tom could feel the singing was becoming infectious. He began to join in, although he didn't see the point in raising his hands as he sang.

We are standing on holy ground,
And I know that there are angels all around.
Let us praise . . . Jesus now!
We are standing in his presence on holy ground.

Everyone looked peaceful and happy. If he hadn't been standing, Tom thought he could doze off. Then Tom noticed someone he vaguely recognized on the other side of the room. It was a woman – an instructor from the English Department. Gloria something-or-other. She waved enthusiastically when she saw Tom and slowly wound her way over to Tom through the crowd.

"Hi. Nice to see you," she said in between the selections of songs they were singing. "I didn't think I'd see anybody from the university *here*. Where do you go to church?"

"St. Albans," Tom replied.

"I used to go to St. Albans!" Gloria something-or-other said excitedly. "Now some of us St. Albans alumni go to the Church in the Fields. It's so . . ." she continued. "Oh, I can't explain it. The Presence is just so strong there, and Kevin – Pastor Kevin Dykes – is just so, ohhhh," she sighed. "I can't explain exactly what it's like. You have to be there and *feel* the Presence of the Holy Spirit." Gloria raised both her hands and sighed with a big smile as the next song began.

> *Seek ye first the kingdom of God*
> *And its righteousness,*
> *And all these things will be given unto you,*
> *Al-le-lu, alleluia.*

Tom could see Bishop Blessing up on the platform with the singers, but off to the side. He looked to Tom unlike either of the two visiting bishops he had seen at St. Albans during the last five years. The bishop was dressed in what looked to be dark Levi's with a wide black belt sporting a large fish symbol buckle. He wore a large ostentatious gold cross on a chain around his neck over a red clerical shirt and white round collar. He was smiling and singing the songs along with everyone else, and occasionally he raised one hand during a song.

> *You are the potter; I am the clay.*
> *Mold me and make me, this is what I pray.*
> *Change my heart, Oh God,*
> *Make me ever true.*
> *Change my heart, Oh God.*
> *Make me be like you.*

Tom glanced at his watch and was shocked to see that he had been standing in the room singing and talking to Gloria for over forty-five minutes, and he had come in late at that. That was nearly the length of an entire service at St. Albans. "Where had the time gone?" Tom thought to himself. It all seemed so effortless. At last the music didn't stop, exactly. It simply trailed off quietly and softly.

"Today is December 5, the feast day of St. Nicholas," Bishop Blessing began, "but nothing reliable is known about a St. Nicholas, in fact he may never have existed, and he may come to us today as a pious fiction. So, I'm not going to talk about St. Nicholas. I'm going to talk about Jesus, and I'm going to talk about myself."

"I've been a bishop a long time, but most of those years I wasn't myself. I mean I just wasn't myself. I went to seminary and became a priest in an ideal parish and married an ideal wife and had three ideal children. Then a big advancement came, and I became a bishop in a more or less ideal place in a diocese filled with beautiful islands in the Caribbean and year-round sun."

"But it wasn't ideal for me," Bishop Blessing continued, "because I was a hypocrite. I knew it, and I was an unhappy hypocrite at that. Oh, I guess I believed in God back in those days to some extent. He was out there *somewhere,* and I probably believed that someone named Jesus thought he was dying for all of mankind two thousand years ago. But it didn't seem right. It didn't *feel* right to me."

"I hated my job, and I really didn't like the people in my diocese. I drank too much. Then I got into narcotics. Then I really got depressed and drank a whole lot more. Then one day everything was gone. My marriage was gone. My wife had taken the children, and they were gone. There had been a turn of Caribbean local politics and even my diocese was suddenly gone. I was a bishop without a flock. And I was broke."

"No Episcopal parish or diocese wanted an alcoholic agnostic bishop without a flock. Finally, a little – no, let's call it tiny – parish in Idaho invited me to come. Although I was supposed to act as an Assistant Priest, there wasn't a lot for me to do other than just hang out, and I did. I was grateful for the job, but oh was I bitter! Did I ever hate the world and what I had become. I don't think I believed at that point that God was even 'out there' any longer. I certainly didn't think he had done me any favors if he were."

"These Rocky Mountain rural people in the tiny parish – they were well meaning, but I must say I thought of them as real hicks. What I hated most was that they were constantly putting their hands on my shoulder and asking if they could pray for me. I thought it was an attack of the zombies. I said no. 'No way' as a matter of fact. They were invading my personal space, and I just wanted to be left alone."

"Then one day after they had hassled me and bugged me to my utmost limits, I told a group of them 'O.K., go ahead and pray for me.' I thought to myself, 'Let's get this ordeal over with.' A group of four or five of them had come to me for the umpteenth time in the parish hall, and I let them gather around me while I sat in a chair, and I let them put their hands on my back and shoulders as they prayed."

"It was the strangest thing," Bishop Blessing said. "I can't remember them praying for anything in particular other than my 'healing'. 'What do I need to be *healed* of?' I thought as they were praying. Then I thought of my perfect life and the perfect shambles I had made of it. A tear started to roll down my cheek and I began to think, 'No, I can't let these people see me cry,' but before I had even fully articulated this thought in my mind I heard a voice speak to me. As God is my witness, I heard the voice of Jesus Christ. I had never heard it before, but it was distinct, and it was clear. It was him all right."

" 'Just let go,' Jesus said to me. 'Let go of the booze. Let go of the dope. Let go of your divorce. Let go of your failures. Let go of your bitterness. Let go of everything. *Just let go*, and I will catch you as you fall.' "

At that moment in the bishop's story, a peculiar and totally unexpected thing happened to Tom Schmidt as he stood listening. Later, he would never be able to describe it sufficiently enough to be understood clearly by others. Later, he would not even be able to recall what Bishop Blessing had said in the next few moments, and it was possible that Tom had not heard it in the first place. The last thing Tom clearly remembered the bishop saying was "Jesus said to me, 'Let go of everything. *Just let go*, and I will catch you as you fall.' " In that moment when perhaps the bishop was braced to describe to his *ad hoc* congregation a life-changing conversion experience that drew him close to God – Tom Schmidt himself experienced the most profound, the most mystical, and the most inexplicably life-changing event of his entire thirty-three years.

In an instant air rushed into Tom's lungs, filling them to a never before experienced capacity. It was as if an atom had suddenly emitted a burst of radiation and he himself was that burst of radiation. It was as if he were transfixed with tweezers like an insect by God and then ran through by God with a mounting pin of spiritual and electrical energy. He thought he was in a kind of cardiac arrest. He thought he had momentarily stopped breathing – had lost the capacity to breathe, but he had not.

Then a total calm and peace came *completely* over Tom. It was the most exhilarating sense of joy and happiness Tom had ever felt. He was delirious with joy. He was beyond himself. He could feel the Holy Spirit coursing through his veins. It was a physical sensation. His mind was not involved. It was his body. It was his heart. It was the Prayer of the Heart. God was a part of him, and he could feel God inside him.

Tom felt like shouting for joy – and he did. He felt like raising his hands in jubilation – and he raised them. He began to say over and over again "Thank you, Jesus! Thank you, Jesus!" He didn't know if he had interrupted the bishop's talk or not, and he didn't care.

Then suddenly Bishop Blessing was off the stage and standing beside him – no, the bishop was embracing Tom with both arms as the bishop shouted "Hallelujah!" and Tom wept openly with tears of happiness and relief and exhilaration all at once. The conference participants gathered around Tom and the bishop and put their arms around them both and joined their voices in peels of "Praise God!" and "Hallelujah!" The Divine Lights climbed back up onto the stage and began to play again. Everyone in the hugging, smiling, crying, shouting, praising and hand-raising group began to sing with them.

> *Lord, you are more precious than silver.*
> *Lord, you are more costly than gold.*
> *Lord, you are more beautiful than diamonds,*
> *And nothing I desire compares to you.*

When the bishop had resumed his position on the stage and was singing with the group, Gloria something-or-other came over to Tom, gave him a Kleenex to wipe his eyes and blow his nose. Then she hugged Tom herself.

"You have the anointing of the Holy Spirit, Tom," she said. "You need to be worshipping with us at the Church in the Fields."

Tom stayed standing in the little meeting room until the last song had been sung, the Divine Lights were packing up their musical instruments and almost everyone else had left the Ball Room. He had been mostly standing in the same general area for over three hours, but he was not the slightest bit tired. On the drive home he turned off the heater and rolled down the driver's side window on his Volvo, letting the frigid night air blow into his face. He sang all of the songs he could remember that had been sung that evening and shouted to the night air many times "Thank you, Jesus! Thank you, Jesus!"

"Quiet, you'll wake the children," Sueann said as Tom opened the living room door singing, "Seek ye first the kingdom of God . . ."

"Are you crazy?" she asked him with a quizzical look on her face.

"Yes, yes," Tom said with a huge smile. "I'm crazy. I'm crazy with the Uncreated Light. The Uncreated Light has entered my heart and driven me crazy with the love of God."

Chapter Five

There was no doubt about it. From his wife and closest colleagues to the most casual observer, Tom Schmidt had changed and seemingly changed overnight. Never a particularly exuberant or outgoing man, Tom became – well, exuberant and outgoing. On the morning of December 6 following his Advent Awakening experience Tom physically awoke with a broad smile on his face and it remained there. He laughed freely and seemed to genuinely enjoy talking to everyone, from the mailman to students on campus.

Moreover, it was not just Tom's attitude that had changed. The *content* of his communications was now markedly different. In some fundamental way Tom now *understood*. He understood the root of virtually all unhappiness. He understood the solution to virtually all physical pain and emotional suffering. He understood the key to successful relationships, careers, personal fulfillment, public service, parenting, and most of the world's problems. Indeed, as a historian he now understood in a profound way the single driving force – both the attraction and the aversion – behind all wars and human struggles and political movements the human race had ever experienced in its history. In a word, the key explanation, the solution, the driving force, and the all to end all problems was "Jesus." It had seemed so simple, really, once Tom understood it.

Moreover, in his own mind Tom now ardently believed that his initial feelings about prayer in general and Prayer of the Heart in particular had been spectacularly proven correct at the Advent Awakening. Without a doubt Tom knew that the Uncreated Light of the Holy Spirit had entered his body *physically* as he was listening to Bishop Blessing, and it had been the greatest experience of his life. The Holy Spirit had brought peace and healing and – yes – even a feeling of ecstasy. Tom was sure his experience was one and the same as had been written about by and concerning the Desert Fathers.

The Holy Spirit had brought Tom a profound knowledge. He had heard that some street drugs were so addicting that a single dose of them brought such a degree of pleasure to the users that the users forever craved additional doses as the single driving force in their lives. The Uncreated Light of the Holy Spirit was far more invigorating and fulfilling than the intoxication of narcotics could ever be, but still Tom understood how the dope addict must feel in the presence of those powerful drugs. Tom wanted more of the Holy Spirit. He wanted it more frequently and in larger doses. He wanted to share his blessings with the world. Everyone had the right and the intended destiny to receive the Uncreated Light.

The Wednesday following Tom's Advent Awakening experience marked the final lecture in the semester prior to the final examination for his *History of Western Civilization: Part One* class. This was a freshman level survey class, and the 114 class-member count was so large that the sessions were held in the O'Neal Auditorium on the other side of the university quadrangle from the College of Liberal Arts building. About ten minutes before the end of class after Tom had finished discussing the implications of the Battle of Culloden in Scotland in 1746, he closed his class lecture notebook at the podium and looked out into the crowded auditorium of freshmen.

"Ladies and gentlemen," Tom began, "the Battle of Culloden concludes our consideration of the first part of Western Civilization and our course of studies in this class. I will be available in Room 202 in the History Department corridor at Allen Hall on Thursday and next Monday from 9 to 11:30 in the morning for any clarification questions about the material we have considered, but not with regard to the nature of questions on the final examination. That will be simply a one hundred question multiple-choice exercise dealing with the time period *only* from the fall of Constantinople through today's lecture. Including the bonus question, it will count for 35% of your grade and will be averaged in with the other two tests this semester for your final grade."

"What I would like to leave you with as a final word this semester," Tom continued, "deals very much with Western Civilization but will not be on the test. Western Civilization was shaped and created by men and women. However, men and women were themselves shaped and created by a much greater force than either time or history. That force was God. Right now, and in this auditorium, God is working with each of our hearts to mold us into the men and women who will, in turn, mold Western Civilization in the immediate future. Through our lectures this semester you have seen examples of those figures in history who accepted the hand of God in their lives and examples of those who did not. Each of you has a choice. I was presented with the same choice recently and I said 'yes' to God. I said 'yes' to God's shaping and molding of my life, and I must tell you that my personal 'yes' to God was the most important affirmation I have ever made and ever will make as long as I live. It is my prayer for each of you that in the beating of your own hearts each of you will likewise say 'yes' to God and follow his prompting of your life journey into the future. If you do, then students at this great university may very well be reading about you a hundred years from now in the "*History of Western Civilization: Part Two.*"

Tom stared into the faces of the auditorium smiling broadly. There were a few seconds of indecisive silence. Then two, and then five, and then twenty-five students began to applaud. Then the entire group seemed to be applauding, and multiple students stood up as the ovation continued. As Tom walked across the quadrangle toward his office in Allen Hall after class, a young man with an arm full of books ran up from behind him.

"Professor Schmidt!" the young man shouted. "Oh, Professor Schmidt!"

"Yes," Tom said smiling after he had stopped and turned around.

"I just wanted to say," stammered the young man as he tried to catch his breath. "I just wanted to say thanks for those words of inspiration you gave us in class today. I appreciated that. I think we all did – even the ones who snickered."

"Oh, don't worry about the snicker people!" Tom replied, laughing. "They'll come around. If a hard head like me can come around, *anybody* can come around. What's your name?"

"Bud," the young man said. "Bud Wolcott."

"Nice to meet you, Mr. Wolcott," Tom said extending his hand to shake the young man's. "Good luck on your final."

Back at his office Tom threw his lecture notebook onto the empty desk against the wall behind his own and turned on his word processor. When the composition program appeared in a green outline on the screen he began to type:

Memorandum
To: Professor Tyler Van Derveer
*   Chair, Faculty Senate*
*   Department of Ag. Economics*
*   School of Agriculture*

From: Tom Schmidt
*   Department of History*
*   Allen Hall, Room 202*

Date: December 8, 1986

Re: Upcoming Faculty Senate Meeting

Dear Tyler:

At our Faculty Senate Meeting over the Christmas break I would like to propose a motion to amend the University Constitution so as to provide that before each committee meeting of the Faculty Senate and prior to any General Assembly of the Senate that intercessory prayers be offered for all the students of the University and any particular student with needs that have been drawn to the attention of any professor or instructor then present and wishing to make intercession. Drawing all of our attention to the Mission Statement contained in the Student Handbook, the salutatory goal of Harvest Christian University is to "foster a distinctly New Testament atmosphere for morally committed students to complete their studies in higher education within a Godly environment." It is inconceivable to me that a "Godly environment" can exist in this institution without prayer taking on a more fundamental role in caring for our young people as opposed to simply being relegated to formal assemblies and graduation ceremonies.

I know some of our colleagues are of a more worldly disposition and will guffaw at this suggestion, but I can assure you others will not. This is a private Christian University and we owe it to our students, their sacrificing parents, and our benefactors to act like it. Please let me know mechanically what I need to do to get this item on the agenda in time for consideration. I am at extension 445.

Tom

On the weekend before final exams, Tom arrived at his office at Allen Hall carrying a large cardboard box. Inside the box was a matted and framed print of William Hunt's "*Light of the World*", a wooden Celtic cross, a New International Study Bible, a rolled paper poster, two nails and a hammer. He hung the framed print showing Jesus holding a lantern and knocking at a garden gate on the wall over the empty desk in his office, and over his own desk he hung the cross. On the outside of his office door, he rolled out and taped down the poster depicting a large hand with the index finger pointing up to a cross at the top of the poster. Below the hand were the words, "Jesus Christ, the one and only way." Inside his office he closed the door and knelt down beside his desk.

"Lord," he prayed. "May I ever be a visible instrument of your love to students and colleagues alike."

In fact, already Tom was becoming somewhat of a sensation in the School of Liberal Arts with students and his colleagues alike. To some students Tom was a bit of a hero. To others he was a religious nut case. His colleagues were generally embarrassed and uncomfortable at Tom's seemingly newfound religiosity, but at the same time Tom was so amiable and friendly that most of his colleagues thought it would have been rather shabby to openly make fun of him. Moreover, when the rumor circulated that Tom was willing to pray with any of his colleagues who felt the disposition or need for prayer, he was actually visited by two instructors privately before Christmas who asked for his prayers and advice.

During the Christmas semester break and a few days before the Faculty Senate meeting, Tom received a short note in the campus mail from Professor Tyler Van Derveer. It read:

Memorandum
To: *Associate Professor Tom Schmidt*
             Allen Hall, Room 202

From: *Tyler Van Derveer*

Re: *Upcoming Faculty Senate Meeting & Yours of 12/8*

Date: *January 3, 1987*

Tom,

Chancellor Post has requested that we hold up on presenting your intercessory prayer proposal to the Faculty Senate until he has had a chance to chat with you. He's in the office Tuesdays and Wednesdays, or you can ring him up at extension 132. Keep me in the loop as to what comes out of your meeting. Interesting proposal!

All the Best, Tyler

On Tuesday, which was actually *the* day before the Faculty Senate meeting, Tom was finally led into Chancellor Homer Post's office in the gothic red brick and twin spired Administration Building by the Chancellor's secretary Biddy Bird. The Chancellor sat behind a large and seemingly ancient carved oak desk situated over a pale blue and white oriental wool rug. Along one of the oak paneled office walls was a dark brown leather divan over which hung 19th Century Italian painter Ferde's "*Christ Emerging from the Tomb.*" Tom had seen the painting before, and he had always thought it was entirely possible the painting was the original Ferde. On the opposite wall hung a large hand-carved alabaster cross adorned with the Triumphant Jesus extending outstretched arms, below which was a cherry wood table with an oriental looking vase containing deep green evergreens and several red carnations. In front of the Chancellor's desk sat two heavy looking leather armchairs matching the divan.

"Tom, Tom!" the Chancellor said enthusiastically as he rose from behind the desk, "Come in, come in! Have a seat. How the heck are you?"

Tom stepped in front of one of the leather chairs and shook Chancellor Post's outstretched hand from across the desk.

"I'm fine, Chancellor Post," Tom said smiling. "Very fine as a matter of fact."

"Homer," replied the Chancellor. "Call me Homer. How about a cup of coffee?"

"No thanks," said Tom.

"Biddy, dear," said the Chancellor holding out his blue patterned china cup and saucer to the secretary. "About half, but don't half my sugar fix."

"Tom," continued the Chancellor settling back into his chair, "Professor Van Derveer shot over a copy of your prayer proposal for the Faculty Senate, and I think it's wonderful and really something we all ought to pray about and work towards."

"Pray about a prayer proposal?" asked Tom.

"Darned right!" replied the Chancellor. "Pray about everything, I always say. 'Pray without ceasing' the Apostle wrote to the Thessalonians."

Biddy Bird came in with the Chancellor's coffee, and before taking a sip he took a minute to stir it mindfully with the silver spoon that had been laid alongside the cup by the meticulous secretary.

Setting the cup and saucer down on the inlaid leather desktop, the Chancellor continued, "Tom, I am totally behind you on this prayer thing, but I want you and I to hold off on presenting it to the Faculty Senate just yet."

"Why hold off?" Tom asked.

"Not by desire, I'll tell you for sure," replied the Chancellor. "It's down and dirty faculty politics, pure and simple. Oh, I don't know why I ever took this job in the first place ten years ago. If it's not sweet-talking the trustees and potential benefactors, it's keeping the faculty from choking each other in open revolt. You remember that 'no smoking on campus thing' two years ago that Martha Kittingslee tried to push through? I thought I would end up losing half of the math department before it all settled down." The Chancellor took another sip of coffee.

"Ah, Tom," continued the Chancellor, "I'll be truthful with you. I just can't risk this prayer deal blowing up into another big mess in the Faculty Senate right now with a bunch of hotheads threatening to walk out right just as the semester is starting. The trouble is not with Liberal Arts. If it was up to your school, we would have all been praying long ago. But the sciences are a different matter. Slots in chemistry and physics are very competitive for us, and several of these guys think we are already too goofy religious-wise for their Darwinesque sensitivities. They will object that we are trying to turn the Faculty Senate into some kind of holy roller camp meeting." The Chancellor searched Tom's face for a reaction.

"Tom," asked the Chancellor, "are you O.K. with that? Can we hold off on the prayer proposal for a while?"

"Sure," said Tom somewhat dejectedly. "If you say it will hurt the university . . ."

"I'm not saying it will actually *hurt the university*," the Chancellor interrupted. "Please don't think that. I know it would be *good* for the university. Just, not yet. Not now. Are you O.K. with that?"

"I'm O.K. with that," replied Tom. "It wasn't my proposal in the first place. It was the Holy Spirit's. We'll just let the Holy Spirit work it out."

"And hopefully soon," said the Chancellor rising and extending his hand out to Tom. "Tom, it was delightful chatting with you. Come by more often! I need this kind of feedback from the faculty."

Chapter Six

Over the next few Sundays Tom found that the services at St. Albans had actually lost some of their appeal to him in ways that he could not altogether put his finger on. The first thing that seemed different was his appreciation of the music. He had always enjoyed the 17th, 18th and 19th Century pipe organ and choral selections played at St. Albans. However, now on Sundays he found himself longing for and actually mentally singing the verses of the simple child-like songs of the Advent Awakening Event even as the organist was playing a musical selection during the communion ceremony.

Another point that seemed odd to Tom was how the pastor, Father Brickwood, had changed over a relatively short period of time. Tom had always thought the priest's sermons were erudite, often clever, and always subtle in their moral implications. Just the kind of sermon a well-educated congregation would seemingly appreciate. But lately Father Brickwood had seemed dour in church, and perhaps even depressed.

"Let's sit closer to the front," Tom whispered to Sueann one Sunday as the couple walked through the huge red oak gothic-looking doors of St. Albans.

"But we always sit *here*," Sueann had mildly complained, nodding to a pew near the back of the sanctuary.

"I'm worried about Father Brickwood," Tom whispered. 'I want to get up close – right up front – so that I can see him better and pray for him while he preaches."

"Oh Tom!" Sueann had said lowly bowing her head and looking furtively around. "Not right up front. No one sits in the first few pews except at Christmas and Easter!"

"Come on!" Tom had whispered. "It's not going to kill you," and to Sueann's slight embarrassment Tom led the couple to the very first pew in the front on the side near the lectern. Being in the first row, Tom and Sueann – the only people seated in the row – did not even have access to kneelers in front of them, and they were forced to kneel all the way down on the carpeted floor during the general confession, the prayers of the people, and the Eucharist service. When Father Brickwood advanced to the lectern for the sermon, he seemed to notice the couple seated in the row immediately below him for the first time. With a quick glance the priest gave them a half smile and then turned to the dozen or so note cards he produced from his alb.

"A preacher in a small country church," Father Brickwood began, "once delivered a fiery sermon on the necessity of forgiving one other. At the conclusion of the sermon he asked everyone in the congregation to bow their heads and pray that they forgive all their enemies. After the prayer he asked for a show of hands from all the people who had forgiven their enemies that morning. The entire congregation raised their hands except a little old ninety-two-year-old woman, the veritable paragon of virtue of the entire group, sitting out front. The preacher was shocked and not a little indignant. 'Bessie,' he blurted out loud, 'don't tell me that at your age you haven't made some enemies?' The old woman replied, 'Nope! I just outlived all of the son of a guns!' " There was scattered laughter in the congregation.

"In the lesson and the Gospel selection for today," Father Brickwood continued, "the invaluable advice to all with ears is focused – not on forgiving *others* – but rather on forgiving ourselves. We are all aware of the 'nasty bit of unpleasantness,' as the expression writer Dorothy Sayers coined, in failing to forgive ourselves. Our sins pollute the world, but we have to go on. We have to tell ourselves, 'yes, we will go on'. Yet, in order to continue notwithstanding the realization of our individual and collective shortcomings, we have to forgive ourselves. In daily inspiration to accomplish this task we ought not overlook the fact that God really, truly has spoken to his people over time. The Bible recounts a contrite Cain and King David and Peter and Mary Magdalene and even Paul all taking counsel with the Lord in their respective times of introspection and emerging from their despair with great insight."

"'But how do we converse with God?' you ask," Father Brickwood continued. "There are many ways to converse with God. God has spoken to me my entire adult life. Some people have found so-called coincidences that happen in their lives not to be coincidences at all when interpreted by faith. As a person prays, his eyes may fall on a particular passage of the Bible that seems to answer his questions and desire for self-forgiveness. A friend or relative may give timely advice – advice which reinforces convictions raised in one's own human heart and mind. We can't all be like the ancient Prophets in the Old Testament who actually heard the voice of God audibly speak to them when they prayed. However, as in the case of the Prophets, we must nevertheless endeavor to see God's hand in our day-to-day activities and hear God's voice through a variety of modes in which he may be speaking to us. We will never be free of guilt from our own polluting sin until we hear God's voice in some way."

As Father Brickwood spoke, Tom became convinced the priest was troubled and very probably because of unanswered prayer in his own life. He looked miserable to Tom as he preached, and the priest periodically gave furtive glances in the direction of Tom and Sueann during his sermon as if *he knew* that *Tom knew* he was in personal torment. Tom ardently prayed that Father Brickwood would be blessed and forgiven for whatever secret sin appeared to be haunting him.

As Tom listened to Father Brickwood and looked up at him with a smile of compassion and understanding, he began to half-expect the priest to suddenly rip his ecclesiastical robe and shirt up the middle and expose the letter "A" carved into his chest by a letter opener.

Tom closed his eyes, raised one hand high over his head and began to pray silently to himself, "No, Lord, don't let Father Brickwood do it. May he stop confessing his own sins to *us*, and just *let go* with the knowledge you will catch him in your arms as he falls." He so wanted Father Brickwood to be happy.

In the midst of his prayer, Tom suddenly became aware that Father Brickwood had stopped talking and the entire congregation was silent. He opened his eyes to see the cleric staring coldly and disapprovingly down at him from the lectern overhead. Tom quickly pulled his hand down into his lap.

"Let the words of my mouth, and the meditation of my heart, be always acceptable in thy sight, O Lord, my strength and my redeemer –

amen," Father Brickwood concluded, sticking his small stack of note cards back into his alb pocket and turning to walk towards the altar. Sueann elbowed Tom in the ribs and moved her head closer.

"What are you do-ing!" she whispered in an exasperated voice. "They'll kick us out of this place."

After church, the couple changed clothes and settled down in their den to read the Sunday newspaper as the boys drove their matchbox cars and trucks over and under the coffee table with sound effects.

"Here's an interesting article," Sueann said from behind the Community News section of the paper: "*New Church Raises Prayers and Vegetables in the Corn Fields*. Do you want me to read it?"

"Sure," said Tom half-interestedly from behind the Sports page.

> *"There's more than corn that is being raised these days at the Green Wave-Clinton crossroads north of Madisonville. A new Christian congregation, The Church in the Fields, has taken up residence in an abandoned barn and silo and is attracting area-wide attendance."*

"I've heard of that church," Tom said interrupting and suddenly giving Sueann his full attention. "I may even know someone who goes there."

"Do you want me to continue reading?" Sueann asked.

"Yes," said Tom.

"Then let me read without interruption, please," she replied.

> *"Shepherded by Reverend Kevin Dykes, the group calls itself the Children of Yahweh, a name stemming from their belief that the Christian church as set forth in the Bible's New Testament never envisioned doing away with any of the Old Testament's religious holidays. 'The biblical evidence simply does not exist,' said Reverend Dykes, 'that Jesus Christ taught we should do away with all of the meaningful holidays God had ordained for his people in the 4,000 odd years predating the birth of our Lord. Jesus was a Jew. All of his disciples were Jews, and all of the first Christians before the Apostle Paul's missionary work were Jews. The Gospels recount that Jesus*

carefully observed all of the important Jewish holidays from the time he was a boy until his death – and so should we. You'd have to come worship with us over time to receive the complete teaching, but I can demonstrate that each and every Jewish holiday mentioned in the Old and New Testaments were in reality precursors of and foreshadowed the coming of Jesus.' The group carries this belief to the point of conducting its weekly worship services on Saturdays in deference to the Seventh Commandment to 'Remember the Sabbath Day and keep it holy.'

Reverend Dykes hails from Minnesota where he earned a Doctorate in Divinity degree from the Minnesota School of Evangelism. He was formerly affiliated as an assistant pastor with the First Assembly of God Church in Brainerd, Minnesota, and then for sixteen years he pastored his own church in St. Paul. When asked what led him to relocate to our community in Iowa, Reverend Dykes replied, 'Prayer and the perfect will of God – pure and simple. When God tells you to move, you have to move no matter how well situated or ostensibly happy you are.

Although the congregation does not utilize its barn and silo for corn production, it does actually grow things. On an adjoining three-acre plot of ground, volunteers from the church grow fruit and vegetables for Madisonville's Meals for the Poor Program as well as for the Food Bank. Additionally, the group operates a nominal-fee day care center for working mothers, and an Iowa State Certified adoption service under the auspices of its Give Life a Chance Ministry for pregnant women. For more information interested persons can call 897 . . ."

"Well," said Sueann, "we're obviously not interested, but . . ."

"But we might be interested," said Tom interrupting her. "Sounds like an interesting place to visit."

"Tom Schmidt," replied Sueann, "that does not sound like an interesting place to visit. The story is interesting, but let's leave it at that. We are Episcopalians. We are happy Episcopalians. There is no need in the world for us to be visiting other churches, whether or not the priest there has some kind of theory about Jewish holidays." Sueann paused a moment. "We're both agreed about that – right?"

"Oh sure, right," replied Tom. "Sueann," he added. "Does the article have a picture? If so, I'd like to see it."

Sueann folded the page back and handed it over. The picture under the headline and framed by the article showed an enormous white barn with an adjacent fifty-foot high wooden cylindrical silo around which metal bands, or hoops, were fastened. The gray-shingled roof appeared new, although the barn itself was of a design from early in the Twentieth Century and needed a coat of paint. Protruding from the roof about halfway up its expanse were two dormer windows, and a huge white canvas or plastic rectangular banner stretched from one window to the other and perhaps ten feet down the roof. It proclaimed, "Church in the Fields – Where God is More Real Than Reality." Although the barn and silo took up most of the picture, Tom could see glimpses in the photograph of vegetable gardens on two sides of the building.

That evening, Tom awoke shortly before midnight and tossed and turned for the better part of an hour before getting out of bed and putting on a robe and slippers. In the darkened den he sat on the divan near the fireplace and prayed.

"Why, Lord," he prayed to himself. "Why can I not feel the Uncreated Light of the Holy Spirit all of the time? I felt it, but now it's gone. I want to feel your presence all of the time."

There was total silence within Tom's mind and no feeling of any presence coursing through his veins as he had felt at the Advent Awakening last year. Actually, the last time he had known for sure that the Uncreated Light was in his heart was when he had prayed with the two instructors who had visited him – separately – in his office before New Year's.

One of the instructors, Merle Banks from the Department of Social Ministry, had talked with Tom about his own struggles being a Christian in what he considered a less than complete Christian University environment. Merle had asked Tom to pray with him to receive the strength to witness to a particularly obdurate full professor in his department. The two men had held hands during the prayer, and Merle had chanted in a special prayer language and wept as he spoke. Suddenly, during the prayer time with Merle, Tom had again felt the hot coursing of the Uncreated Light pulsing through his chest and arms and even in his hands holding on to Merle's. Moreover, the feeling had not been all that transitory. He had felt he was wonderfully alive and refreshed for three or four days after that.

Tom wondered if there was something he was doing – or perhaps something that he was not doing – that was retarding the flow of the Uncreated Light into his heart recently. He worried whether he had somehow inadvertently dampened the flow of the Holy Spirit within his heart – perhaps by agreeing with Chancellor Post not to propose the prayer amendment at the Faculty Senate. Had God wanted him to press the issue? He wished he could know God's will directly and not through suppositions and abstract feelings.

Although he had not recalled it, he wondered if the copy of the New International Study Bible he kept at home had a reference to the "Uncreated Light" in the index where he could read more on it directly in the Bible or whether that term was a description first used by the Desert Fathers. He walked in the dark into his little office adjacent to the foyer and turned on the light. The office had apparently been recently straightened up by Sueann, and everything was back in its place. The Bible was on a shelf over the desk.

As Tom reached over his desk to pull the Bible from the shelf, the Bible fell from his grasp down to the surface of the desk and upon the picture of his father with a loud crash – sending the picture and the Bible down to the floor.

"Tom," he heard Sueann's voice from the bedroom. "Are you all right?"

"Yeah, Sue," Tom answered. "I'll be in, in a minute."

Bending over to retrieve the picture – now with a cracked glass – and the Bible, Tom saw that the book had fallen open at the binding. Tom pulled the Bible up to the desktop still open at the place and laid it down. His eyes instantly fell upon a verse on the left-hand page. It was Deuteronomy 5:12: "*Observe the Sabbath day and keep it holy, as the Lord your God commanded you.*"

Chapter Seven

During the next week, Tom thought more and more about the Church in the Fields, and he frequently recalled Gloria something-or-other's comment at the Advent Awakening that one could "feel the Presence of the Holy Spirit" during the services. He wondered if the "presence" described by Gloria was the same experience he and the Desert Fathers referred to as the "Uncreated Light." It would be, Tom thought, out of the question suggesting a visit to Sueann. She had made that quite clear after reading about the Children of Yahweh in the Sunday paper. But perhaps he could visit the church for its Saturday service and still fully participate with Sueann and the children on Sunday at St. Albans. The more Tom thought about it the more he became convinced that his attending just a service or two at the Church in the Fields would undoubtedly rejuvenate his connection with God. He could recharge his batteries, and Sueann would not even have to know. A small diversionary excuse would protect her from needlessly becoming upset. He called the number in the newspaper article he had rescued from the trash and verified the Church in the Field's location and time of Saturday service.

"Sueann," Tom said the next Saturday morning while pouring himself a second cup of coffee in the couple's kitchen, "I need to work this morning and probably the next few Saturday mornings on my new book at the University's library. I have a publishing deadline coming up if I am going to be able to use the University Press to print the thing. I can be back by two."

"Does that mean the grass is not going to get mowed today?" Sueann asked.

"No, no," answered Tom. "I'll get it taken care of this afternoon, and if not today, tomorrow after church for sure."

"Promises, promises," Sueann said.

Tom finished his coffee and kissed Sueann on the cheek on his way out of the door.

Tom drove out of town north on Interstate 101 until the Green Wave Road exit and then east on through the cornfields until he got to the Church in the Fields at Clinton Road. As Tom pulled into the church parking lot, he saw several swing sets and a large slide off to one side at which several dozen children played. A large old Bluebird school bus painted white with "Jesus is Lord" emblazoned along the side was parked at the back of the parking lot. There were perhaps two hundred cars, pickups and vans parked in rows on the gravel parking lot, some extending into the uncultivated field immediately to the south of the silo.

As Tom walked toward the huge double doors of the barn-made-church, he saw a large number of people standing in groups chatting outside and enjoying the sunshine before the commencement of the service. Near the door, Tom saw his acquaintance Gloria excitedly wave her hand at him. She ran to meet him and took him by the hand.

"I'm thrilled to see you," said Gloria rapidly. "I prayed that you'd come. Once you have the anointing, the Episcopal Church just seems dead. Anyway, it did for me. Come with me, I want you to meet pastor Kevin. He's inside." Gloria pulled Tom along, through the big doorway and into the cavernous interior of the barn.

Inside, Tom could see where the large floor area of the barn had been paved over with concrete and covered with low-nap red carpeting. Several hundred metal folding chairs were arranged in rows with broad aisles in the center and on the sides. Flooring from what had once been the huge hayloft overhead was removed to expose the cross joists from which hung banners proclaiming slogans of jubilation such as "Hallelujah!" and "I am the Captain of the Hosts saith the Lord God!" Just inside the doorway, Gloria led Tom through a crowd over to a well-dressed man talking and laughing with about a dozen or so people.

"Pastor Kevin," said Gloria pulling Tom up to the minister, "I want you to meet my friend and a colleague from the university, Tom Schmidt. He teaches in the History Department."

"History, eh?" said Reverend Dykes shaking Tom's hand. "Any biblical history?"

"A little," replied Tom hesitatingly. Reverend Dykes appeared to be an athletic and trim man in his early forties with gray accents in his neatly styled dark brown hair. He was clean-shaven and carried a seemingly perpetual broad smile on his face. He wore an expensive-looking light blue Italian silk suit with a neon pink tie and matching pink silk handkerchief displayed from his coat breast pocket. On one of his French cuffs fastened with gold cuff links was the monogrammed initials "KKD", and his fingernails were manicured and coated with a clear polish. The pattern and color of his designer belt, a kind of lizard skin, matched his expensive-looking shoes. He wore a plain gold wedding band, and the well-dressed woman next to him was presumably his wife.

"Welcome, Tom Schmidt!" said Reverend Dykes. "I see you are married. This is my wife Mary Ann. Is your wife here?" Tom shook hands with Mrs. Dykes. She looked to be younger than Reverend Dykes, though how much younger he couldn't say. At least one of the children in the immediate vicinity – a three or four-year-old – was obviously hers and hung on to her left arm, periodically pulling her.

"Don't!" Mrs. Dykes scolded the child after releasing Tom's hand.

"No, not this Sabbath Day," replied Tom. "She had to stay with the children."

"Next time bring her!" Reverend Dykes replied. "We have a nursery, a complete Sabbath School program and Children's Church for the young ones."

Just then music could be heard from the front of the church, and Reverend Dykes excused himself to walk up front.

"Let's sit up front!" said Gloria enthusiastically, guiding Tom down the center aisle. As Tom walked with Gloria down the aisle, Tom could see a five-piece band with three electric guitars, a trumpet and drums stationed in one corner of the floor area to the side of a podium up front. Behind the podium a huge cloth banner suspended by ropes spanned the entire width of the interior of the barn. It proclaimed, "Speak to me Lord, your servant is listening." People streamed into the church from the outside at the sound of the music, and soon the building's interior was filled to capacity as Tom and Gloria stood in a row between two ranks of chairs near the front of the church.

The volume of the music increased substantially, and the tempo livened as well. The drummer rhythmically tapped out a fast-paced beat on a full set of drums, and the base guitar joined in as the lead guitarist picked out a fast rock and roll melody. Three female singers without instruments each stood at a microphone in a line off to one side of the lead guitarist and began to rhythmically clap their hands in unison. In a moment three hundred people were clapping in unison to the fast-paced music.

"People of God!" the lead guitarist yelled into his microphone over the volume of the instruments, the drums, and the clapping. "People of God, let's have church!"

There was a general yell of delight from the crowd and the lead guitarist again rapidly moved his pick over the strings. Then, pushing his guitar dramatically behind him and grabbing the microphone with one hand, he sang.

> *Anything is pos-sible! Any thing is pos-sible!*
> *Anything is pos-ible*
> *With God!*
> *Anything is pos-sible! Any thing is pos-sible!*
> *Anything is pos-ible*
> *With God!*
>
> *You are the heavens in the night,*
> *Your are the brightest morning light,*
> *Your are the reason for my life.*
> *You are the God of strength and might.*

With the beginning of the chorus a second time, the handclapping congregation rose to its feet and joined in. Tom could see where a giant white screen high over the podium was now lit up with the words of the song scrolling down as the song leader played and sang.

> *Anything is pos-sible! Any thing is pos-sible!*
> *Anything is pos-ible*
> *With God!*

Anything is pos-sible! Any thing is pos-sible!
Anything is pos-ible
With God!

As the band kept up the heavy fast beat and the trumpet and guitars played a musical interlude to the song, Tom saw two men in coats and ties running full speed down one of the side aisles, across the front and up the center aisle toward the back of the church. Each man had a white handkerchief in his hand which he waved overhead as he ran. The band leader led everyone through the chorus one more time, and then the band abruptly stopped.

"People of God," said the band leader into the microphone. "We're all blessed to be here together, Praise God! I'm Jerry Jenko, the head of the music ministry here at God's place in the corn fields – Praise God, the Church in the Fields. Let's just bow our heads and enter into worship as one people with one heart and one mind – all for Jesus."

He began to play a slow melody and sang softly into the microphone. The three female singers echoed the lines in unison behind him and held their hands up as they sang with their eyes closed. Soon the entire congregation joined in with their hands held up as the big screen flashed the lyrics overhead.

Oh, Jesus, king above all kings,
Blessed Redeemer, Li-iving Wor-or-ord,
Eman-uel, God is a-mong us,
Beautiful savior, loving Lord.

"Jee sho ho bo kasha," the music minister said into the microphone as he finished. "Thank you Lord. Thank you Jesus."

The music continued for song after song – some selections breathtakingly fast and exhilarating, and some slow and prayerful – with words of encouragement or prayer by the music minister in between many of the selections. During the faster selections both men and women would leave their seats to run down and up the aisles, and during two songs what looked to Tom to be teenage boys and girls – perhaps twenty of them – ran through the aisles carrying large red, green and yellow nylon flags on short poles. After about thirty minutes the song tempos began to consistently be of the slow and prayerful variety. At one point the final song was simply ended, as the band members and the three singers, along with the band leader, fell into silence, bowed their heads, and uttered "Jesus, Jesus," over and over again in soft voices.

Then the entire congregation began to pray quietly in a variety of soft-spoken phrases and a jumble of mysterious and incomprehensible prayer languages. Then, some individuals in the large congregation began to raise their voices, but in a singing tone and quality. Other voices joined in, each in a different meter or tempo as the mysterious prayer languages joined in a louder and louder refrain. What might have been imagined as a rather cacophonous din in fact sounded to Tom as veritably angelic. As the incomprehensible singing continued, a line of people began to form off to the side of the podium in the front of the church, and Reverend Dykes appeared near the head of the line. He held whispered discussions with the people in line one by one as the singing trailed off and various members of the congregation sat quietly down into their folding chairs or kneeled on the carpet in front of their seats. Tom could hear weeping among the congregation, and a few people actually wailed with seeming grief. Beside him, Tom turned to see Gloria kneeling on the carpet in front of her chair with tears flowing down both of her cheeks.

"Gloria!" said Tom. "Are you all right?"

Nodding her head affirmatively, Gloria looked up at Tom through her tears, smiling.

Tom suddenly heard a voice over the church's sound system. He looked up to see the first man who had been in line up front standing at the podium speaking.

"You are my beloved people," the man said. "A people dear to my heart and a royal priesthood. Love, my people. Love each other with undivided and unwavering hearts." The man turned and walked down the steps from the podium.

"Yes!" Tom heard people around him say. "Yes, Lord!" Gloria echoed beside Tom. "Praise God!"

One by one individuals in line came to the podium to speak and return to their seats. Tom noticed that one woman in line was barefoot. When she arrived at the podium she said, "the Lord God has instructed me to say that he dearly loves his people – he will never leave you orphans." Another man threw out his arms and said into the microphone "I am the Lord your God, and you will not have any other gods before me. Thus, I say to you, Brethren, follow your pastor even as my sheep follow their shepherd. Follow my shepherd." Yet another man said at the microphone, "I am getting the message, brothers and sisters, that the Lord is calling us to be more deliberate in our ministry for the unwed mothers of Iowa. I just thought I would share that with you." As other people rose from their chairs and walked to the front, Reverend Dykes continued to hold a whispered discussion with each of them before it was their turns at the podium. Once, a woman waiting to be heard in line returned to her seat after her discussion with Reverend Dykes as another person ahead of her was speaking at the podium.

When the last people wanting to speak had returned to their seats in the congregation, Reverend Dykes reached up to the podium and picked up a large black leather-bound Bible. He walked out into the congregation about ten feet up the center aisle and opened the book that had been marked with a slip of paper.

"Our text for today is from the Sixth Chapter of Luke," said Reverend Dykes, "beginning at the 22nd verse. Open your Bibles and read along with me, Beloved:

> *Blessed are ye, when men shall hate you, and when they shall separate you from their company, and shall reproach you, and cast out your name as evil, for the Son of Man's sake. Rejoice ye in that day, and leap for joy: for behold, your reward is great in heaven: for in the like manner did their fathers unto the prophets.*

"Skip to verse 26," continued Reverend Dykes:

> *Woe unto you when all men shall speak well of you! For so did their fathers to the false prophets.*

"Do you ever get the feeling," said Reverend Dykes closing his Bible, "that you are an oddball as far as the world is concerned? That you just don't fit in? That people snicker behind your back, or worse still to your face? Did you ever start to think that being a Christian is a tough, thankless, un-popular, un-glamorous and un-appreciated thing to be? Did you ever think to yourself that you've lost the ear of your children because you've set too many Godly rules of behavior, and you've lost the respect of your brother-in-law who thinks you're a religious fanatic, and you've even lost the friendship of your neighbors because they want to drink beer at their barbeques and so they have stopped inviting you and the wife over, and anyway you give them the creeps with all of your talking about God! Well, if that has happened to you. If that *is* happening to you. If you are unpopular and outcast and considered square and old fashioned and laughed at because you are some kind of a nut – some kind of a Jesus fanatic, then I say Praise God!"

"You're doing something right. You are acting Christ-like. They laughed at Jesus. They accused Jesus of things he didn't do and crimes he didn't commit and even thoughts that he didn't think. And then they killed him! Well, that's the way it is with us Christians. When everybody starts clapping you on the back and inviting you to their wine and cheese parties and calling you a great Christian – watch out! They didn't invite Jesus to their wine and cheese parties. They spat on him, and then they drove nails first into *this* wrist," he shouted pointing, "and then into *this* wrist and then into *these* feet – and then they hung him on a cross and killed him. When he didn't die quickly enough, they threw a spear into him to finish the job."

"Did you ever feel like that? Did anyone you thought you knew, and you thought was dependable and you thought you even loved, stab you in the back and try to finish you off? Of course, you have. We all have. We all know what it's like to be a Christian and the price we have to pay."

Reverend Dykes continued to preach for over an hour, but to Tom the minutes flew by. It was the most relevant, the most fascinating, and the most poignant sermon he had ever heard. As he spoke and made significant points, individuals in the congregation would shout out "Praise God!" and "Amen to that!"

At the end of the sermon, Reverend Dykes called for the Elders of the church to come forward and if anyone in the congregation needed prayers for healing to likewise come forward and receive it. As people lined up, presented themselves at the front of the church for healing and spoke into the microphone about their special needs, Reverend Dykes would say something about the love of Jesus and the Holy Spirit and then pray in tongues in a mystical prayer language. Some of Reverend Dykes' utterances were short and repetitious like a chant. Others were extensive and seemed to have syntax and structure like a foreign language would appear to have to one not understanding it.

"Shal la la, pente kapasha, oh thank you Jesus, ro sha sha bah, sha sha bah," Reverend Dykes prayed. Reverend Dykes produced a little brass cylindrical container with a screw top that contained what Gloria whispered to Tom was "holy oil." Reverend Dykes dipped a finger into the cylinder and applied it in an oily "sign of the cross" on each healing recipient's forehead. When he laid his hands upon one woman's head, who had said into the microphone that her husband was an atheist and had objected to her coming to the meeting that morning, she fell backwards suddenly, apparently unconscious, and she was lowered to the red carpeted floor by two of the Elders who had moved into position behind her.

"Just let her rest in the spirit there for a while," Reverend Dykes instructed with one hand suspended over her. "A healing spirit is upon her. Ro rash sha sha kasha! In Jesus' name!"

One man, referred to only by the name of "Charlie" hobbled up to the front on a wooden cane. After praying for the man and applying holy oil to his forehead in the sign of the cross, Reverend Dykes suddenly grabbed the cane from the man's hand and threw it against the podium with a loud crash. Yelling into the microphone, he said "Be healed in the name of Jesus of Nazareth and accept the healing balm of the Holy Spirit." Charlie had fallen to the ground on all fours.

"Get up and walk, in the name of Jesus!" Reverend Dykes commanded in a loud voice. "You don't need a crutch. You don't need a cane. Let Jesus be your crutch and your cane!" Then, with seemingly superhuman strength, Charlie pushed himself up to an upright kneeling and then a standing position and walked a straight unsteady path back to his folding chair in the middle of the congregation. The congregation suddenly broke into a general joyful melee with the flags appearing again held by young people running down and up and around the rows of folding chairs. People raised their hands and chanted "Glory to God!" in unison, and men in their places pulled white handkerchiefs from their pockets and waved them overhead. Tom thought to himself that either Reverend Dykes and Charlie were in cahoots and complete charlatans or he had just witnessed firsthand the very hand of God move.

At the coffee hour following the service, Gloria stood with Tom, talking.

"Tom," she said, "when I was praying this morning, God spoke to me and gave me a word of knowledge about you. I don't want to pry, but your wife isn't with you about us – I mean about our church here, is she?"

"No," said Tom. "She isn't."

"I'm sorry," said Gloria taking Tom's hand. "It will work out. You'll see."

"She's tough," said Tom sadly.

"Well, we want her to get un-tough. We want her to get better, don't we? I'll pray for her healing."

"Thanks," said Tom.

Before leaving, Tom filled out a Newcomer Registration Card at a table near the big double doors of the church and dropped it into the small basket provided. For his address, Tom filled in "Room 202, Allen Hall, Harvest Christian University, Madisonville, Iowa 50125."

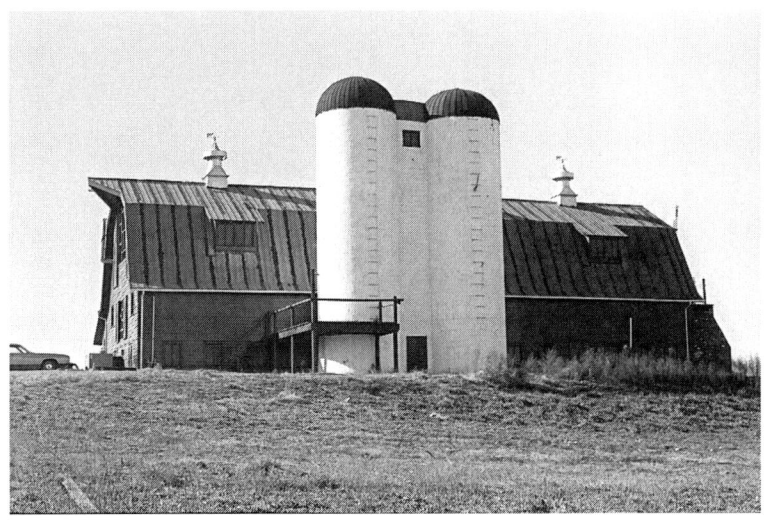

Chapter Eight

"What's up, fellow Christian?" Gloria asked, standing at the open door to Tom's office in the History Department corridor at Allen Hall the following Tuesday.

"Gloria!" said Tom excitedly looking up from his desk. "In fact," he continued shifting through a pile of notes on his desk and coming up with a yellow note pad piece of paper, "Gloria Singleton, Master's Degree Connecticut College, PhD Dartmouth, dissertation, '*Repentance, Judgment & Rejuvenation in John Milton's Paradise Lost,*' 442 Europe Street, Madisonville, single, divorced." Tom's voice trailed off suddenly.

"I'm sorry," said Tom. "I looked you up. I was embarrassed I knew so little about you while you were able to introduce me to Pastor Dykes last Sunday. I didn't mean to be so personal."

"That's O.K., Thomas Alvin Schmidt," Gloria replied, "Master's in History, Iowa State University, PhD, Illinois State, Moline, dissertation, *Wage Differentials Between Conscripted and Volunteer Legionnaires in the Latter Byzantine Empire.* I looked you up, too." Tom and Gloria both laughed.

"You'll never guess," said Gloria, "whose card the Newcomers' Committee gave me to follow up on, seeing as I was a University person."

"I can't imagine," replied Tom. "Was it a person's who was so afraid of his wife's disapproval that he gave his office address on the card?"

"I think it might have been," said Gloria. "How about a cup of coffee?"

"I've got class in a few minutes," said Tom.

"Then how about a quick word of prayer?" asked Gloria.

"Sure," said Tom. "Come in."

Gloria stepped into Tom's cramped office and shut the office door, sliding down into the empty desk chair next to Tom's.

"Tom," said Gloria, "You *are* loved – do you know that?"

"I don't know," said Tom. "I guess I am, but by whom is the question."

"I love you," replied Gloria. "The people at the church love you – your wife loves you. I'm sure of that in my spirit. Give me your hands."

Tom put his hands into Gloria's. Her hands felt incredibly soft, and he could smell her delightful scent from the two or three feet or so separating them.

"Rosh, ka, ka, dee licta, dee licta, rosh," prayed Gloria with her eyes shut tight. "Yes, Jesus. Yes, Jesus."

Rather suddenly, Tom straightened bolt upright in his chair.

"Gloria!" Tom said in an excited whispered voice. "Tee kumba, tee kumba, roshee. Tee kumba roshee!"

Tom felt invigorated and as if a bolt of energy was being shot into his body. The Uncreated Light was back, and with it God had given to him a mystical prayer language all of his own.

"Tee kumba, tee kumba, roshee! Tee kumba roshee!" Tom prayed with eyes wide-open clutching Gloria's hands.

"Oh, yes, Lord Jesus!" Gloria prayed, pulling Tom to her and holding him in her arms as tears dripped down her cheeks. "Anoint your beloved. Anoint your beloved."

In the following weeks, Tom did not limit his visits to the Church in the Fields to "just a service or two" on Saturdays as he had vowed at first. In fact, Tom continued to visit the Church in the Fields with greater and greater involvement in the services himself, and on two occasions he went to the front of the church for prayers after the sermon by Reverend Dykes. On Newcomer's Saturday, Tom was among six people who were called to the front of the congregation by Reverend Dykes and given the handheld microphone to introduce themselves and tell the congregation how the Lord had brought him into their midst. Energized with the Uncreated Light of the Holy Spirit, Tom took the microphone and announced himself to the congregation.

"I am Tom Schmidt and I'm a hypocrite," Tom said. "I didn't have the intellectual or emotional or spiritual guts to become a Christian – never did. I was a coward. The Holy Spirit finally got tired of my procrastination and hardheaded hypocrisy and just zapped me. When I was baptized as a Christian I went, like Nicodemus, and slinked into a little chapel in a big church when no one was looking in order to be privately baptized. I didn't want my atheist friends at the university to know I was a Christian, and I didn't want anybody I met at church to think I hadn't been a Christian for many years by then. I didn't confess any sins because I didn't think I had any sins to confess. After I was baptized, I said my little prayers and sang the church hymns – but I didn't know the Lord Jesus. I didn't know the Holy Spirit. Oh, I was proud! I thought I was so smart. Proud and smart. And I was an intellectual. I read and studied, and I was convinced I had Jesus and Christianity all figured out from an *intellectual* point of view. But I found out that there's nothing intellectual about love, and God didn't love me from an *intellectual* point of view. He doesn't save us from self-destruction '*intellectually*.' No, he gets down with us in our slobber and our tears and in our vomit from too much booze and he takes us in his arms like a lover and he whispers into our ear 'don't worry about all of this. I love you, and that's all that matters.' "

"I didn't love God first," Tom continued. "I used my learning like a shield and kept him away from me. I didn't want that emotional crap you see in church with all the tears and the praise and the hallelujahs. I thought Christians were idiots. I was a smart guy – I had it all figured out, and it hadn't cost me one tear. Then one night, God just couldn't stand it anymore. I know that saying about the 'Patience of Job,' but I also know personally that God got just plain impatient with me and my hypocrisy. One night at a renewal conference when my eyes were glassed over and I stopped up my ears to what was being said for the umpteenth time, God just zapped me anyway. He chased me down and tackled me. He held me there with his arms until I couldn't move any more, and then he whispered into my ear 'there, you dumb German, don't you realize how much I love you?' He kissed me and he hugged me. He replaced my blood with the blood of Jesus, and he replaced my intellectual thoughts with the Uncreated Light of the Holy Spirit. I haven't been the same since, and it's not always easy. It seems, I cry more now in a month than I cried in my entire childhood, but I also laugh more now in one year than I laughed in my whole life before being tackled by the Lord. The hand of the Lord is upon me. I'll never again live the same life as I lived before I knew Jesus. Hallelujah."

The congregation clapped loudly, and several voices were heard shouting "Hallelujah!" Then Tom gestured to give the microphone back to Pastor Kevin, but suddenly Tom jerked the microphone back to his mouth and fell to his knees.

"Tee kumba, tee kumba, roshee, tee kumba roshee!" Tom shouted into the microphone. "I am the Lord your God," Tom said in a deep and commanding voice. "Do not bring me candy and flowers and make me silly compliments as you would a childhood friend, saith the Lord. I am your lover. I am your faithful lover who will never love another more deeply than I love you. Never stray from me. Never be untrue. Love your husbands. Love your wives. But never be deceived. I am the most faithful lover you will ever have!"

A crowd of people from the congregation, mostly women, left their places and rushed forward, falling to their knees in a circle four persons deep around Tom clinging to each other and Tom, shouting, "Lord, Lord!" Several began to weep and wail. One woman near Tom suddenly grabbed his hair in one hand and jerked his head back sharply.

"My God, my God!" the woman screamed.

Reverend Dykes, at first genuinely stunned by the outburst – both of Tom and of the women in the congregation – seemed to compose himself, and he waded through the rows of women to Tom and urged him to stand. As Tom rose to his feet a voice rang out.

"People of God!" yelled a voice from the congregation. It was Gloria Singleton's voice. "I know this Man of God," Gloria shouted above the din of "Hallelujahs" and "Glory to Gods". "I witnessed this man," Gloria continued, "receive the anointing at the Hilton Hotel last December, and it broke my heart in two at the sight. The Living God has told me this man is God's very own anointed prophet!"

A voice suddenly rose from among the women kneeling around Tom and the Pastor.

"This is my adopted child Tom, saith the Lord!" an older woman shouted, "and he will arise with my anointing to become a prophet among my people."

The band began to play a rousing tune, and the teenagers appeared running up and down the broad aisles between the rows of chairs with their flags as the congregation, including the kneeling crowd around Tom and the Pastor, stood again and began to rhythmically clap. Waving his hands to quiet down the congregation, Reverend Dykes spoke.

"God's precious will has spoken," the Reverend said into the handheld microphone. "A word of knowledge has just come to me that this man is indeed one of the very anointed of God. Yes, of God Jehovah Jireh!"

The congregation shouted their approval, and the teenagers again ran through the aisles with the flags as the band began a lively electric guitar and drum heavy chorus of, "*Yes, Lord, Yes Lord, Yes My Lord My God.*"

After the chorus ended, Reverend Dykes again motioned to quiet down the congregation, produced his brass cylinder of holy oil, and unscrewed the lid.

"My brother Tom," said the Reverend into the microphone, "do you accept God's precious will for your life?"

"Yes," said Tom into the microphone.

"Do you renounce the devil, all forms of witchcraft and the forces of the anti-Christ which rebel against God?" the preacher asked.

"Yes," Tom answered with tears beginning to drip down both cheeks. "I renounce *all* of them."

"Do you renounce the corruption of this world which seeks to destroy the people of God?"

"Yes," Tom said.

"Do you renounce all sinful desires that draw you from the love of God?" the Reverend continued.

"I renounce them all," he replied.

"Will you keep the holy days of the Lord in both the Old and the New Testaments, act as an Elder of this church befitting a man of God and a Christian gentleman in all ways and at all time?" Reverend Dykes asked into the microphone.

"I will," said Tom weeping.

"Shal la la, pente kapasha, oh thank you Jesus, ro sha sha bah, sha sha bah," Reverend Dykes prayed into the microphone. "I anoint you Elder and Prophet – one of our very own!"

Reverend Dykes put his thumb into the opened cylinder and marked a cross on Tom's forehead, pushing Tom's head backwards with the palm of his hand. Although Tom did not intend to either lose balance or fall, he did on both counts and threw his arms up as he careened rearward, only to be caught by two Elders who had moved into position behind him.

"I'm all right. I'm all right," Tom said.

"Of course, you're all right, Elder Tom," Reverend Dykes shouted into the microphone. "You have the Holy Spirit as your parachute when you fall!" The congregation laughed with pure joy and began singing, *Yes, Lord, Yes Lord, Yes My Lord My God* again spontaneously. Almost immediately the band began to play and picked up the tempo.

With the anointing of the holy oil Tom once again felt the Uncreated Light of the Holy Spirit enter his heart as if in jolts of electric ecstasy, and he was beside himself with joy.

"You know," Reverend Dykes said as the congregation slowly worked its way back to the seats and Tom wiped his face and nose with a white handkerchief one of the Elders handed him, "the anointed role of prophet is a ministry rife with heart-felt pain and tribulation on behalf of God's people. 'Woe be unto you,' says the Lord, 'If you say unto my people that which I have not instructed you to say, but a double woe unto thee who silently withholds the words I have commanded you to speak.'"

At the coffee hour, Gloria excitedly hugged Tom.

"Now we need to work on your wife," said Gloria with a big smile.

As a new Elder, Tom had been called to the front of the church with the other Elders to pray with those needing healing, and many people stopped by the coffee pot after the service to introduce themselves or give the new Elder a hug.

That night Tom had the most bizarre dream. Sueann was there, and so also was Gloria Singleton. Both of the women were wearing white robes, but when Sueann turned toward him the number "666" was emblazoned on her forehead.

"Do you renounce all forms of witchcraft?" Tom heard the thundering voice of Reverend Dykes ask.

"Yes, Lord," Tom responded.

"Then do not be deceived," the voice rang out. "I, the Lord your God, am the most faithful lover you will ever have!"

Suddenly in the dream Tom's attention changed to Gloria who opened her robe displaying her naked and beautiful breasts. She dropped the garment at her feet. Gloria looked lovely, and her white creamy skin was aglow with the Uncreated Light that Tom could see pulse into and out of her heart as it beat. She reached her right hand out to Tom as if to beckon him over to her.

"Do you renounce all sinful desires that draw you from the love of God?" the Reverend's voice boomed.

"Gloria is not a sinful desire!" Tom shouted. "She is not a sinful desire!"

"Tom! Tom!" Sueann said shaking Tom. "You are having a nightmare. Who is Gloria?"

Tom rose up to a sitting position on the bed and rubbed his forehead. "Nothing. Nobody. A dream," he replied groggily.

Chapter Nine

Despite his telling Sueann he had been working on his new book, "*Post-Modern Trends in Christian History*" every Saturday morning for the previous two months, Tom had made very little progress research-wise, and he had not actually written one word. The only published work of his of any length following his dissertation was "*Striking Comparisons: The Byzantine Transformation to Orthodoxy and the Roman Catholic Counter-Reformation,*" had been warmly received by his colleagues in the College of Liberal Arts, and had led – in part – to his promotion in the History Department to Associate Professor. However, that book had been written over three years ago and in truth and fact the book had actually sold less than two hundred copies. While there was not an official "publish or perish" policy among the various departments of the university at this time, there nevertheless was an unofficial policy expecting associate and full professors to publish on a regular basis, and Tom was over-due to get another project into print.

Tom had originally intended "*Post-Modern Trends in Christian History*" to be a history of the pentecostal movement in American Christian denominations from 1960 onward, and he had accumulated over five hundred research note cards and several dozen books on the subject, all of which he stored in his locked faculty cubical at the university library. However, following his anointing as an Elder and Prophet at the Church in the Fields, Tom totally lost interest in the research track he was pursuing, and in fact there came a point one Tuesday late Fall afternoon that he scooped up all five hundred seventeen of his research cards and his two research notebooks, and threw them into the gray metal trash can beside his desk in his faculty cubical. He went and got a book trolley from the circulation desk and piled up the thirty-two references he had previously pulled from the library shelves and special ordered from inter-library loans onto the trolley, returning it full to the circulation desk.

None of this activity was the least bit counter-productive as far as Tom was concerned. On the contrary, he thought to himself, he was simply clearing his desk and symbolically clearing his mind to begin the *real* work at hand. Indeed, Tom would write "*Post-Modern Trends in Christian History,*" and possibly it would be the greatest book of its kind in the history of the world. The reason for Tom's substantial expectations was that he fully expected the Holy Spirit – the same Holy Spirit that was identified as the ancient third element of the Trinity and one and the same with the Uncreated Light of the Desert Fathers – would *personally* dictate the entire work to him.

For what had happened to Tom in the months following his anointing was perhaps of monumental significance to both him and to the entire world of faith as far as Tom was concerned: Tom had discovered a way to really, truly and without any doubt *communicate with God.*

No, this was not a communication consisting of any of the seven species of "prayer" outlined in the Episcopal *Book of Common Prayer* or by Father Brickwood's beliefs of interpreted coincidences. This was the *real thing*. Words. He talked. The Uncreated Light answered him. God now spoke into his ear and into his mind both at home and at school. When Tom sat at his IBM Word Processor in his office at school, the Uncreated Light would dictate as he typed. The real thing.

"Glory be to God!" Tom would say at his desk.

"Indeed," he would type the words spoken to him. "How was your drive from home today, Tom?"

"Is that you, Lord my God?" Tom would type.

"The Alpha and the Omega – the beginning and the end – the one all to end all," Tom's fingers would type in answer to his question.

Tom had discovered the channel of communication with God almost by accident one Saturday afternoon following services at the Church in the Fields when he had sat drinking a cup of coffee in his office at home. Although Tom had read widely *through* the Bible and was familiar with a great many of its passages, he had never actually read the entire Bible from cover to cover – in context as he assumed it had been laid out historically.

He had purchased a copy of the King James Version of the Bible as an adjunct to his New International Study Edition – not wanting to study the passages as much as savor the Word of God and enjoy it. He had, of course, begun with Genesis, Chapter One, Verse One, and he had been almost instantly struck that the Uncreated Light was present at the very commencement of the existence of creation itself.

"And the Spirit of God moved upon the face of the waters," Verse Two recounted. In the very next verse, a new species of light would flood the universe and indeed all of creation: visible light. But it was clear to Tom that the Uncreated Light was God himself and had been present from the very beginning. The Uncreated Light was the Creator of the visible light of the Sun, the Moon, and the Stars. It was "*un*-created" light because it was the Creator himself – who has no beginning or end. Who *is* the very beginning and the end of all created things.

On this particular long rainy afternoon Tom had progressed through some three hundred pages to the First Book of Samuel, to where the child prophet, a servant of the priest Eli, lies down to sleep in the Temple at Shiloh near the Ark of the Covenant. Tom read:

> [T]he Lord called Samuel; and he answered, Here am I. And he ran unto Eli, and said, here am I; for thou calledst me. And he said, I called not; lie down again. And he went and lay down. And the Lord called yet again, Samuel. And Samuel arose and went to Eli, and said, here am I; for thou didst call me. And he answered, I called not, my son; lie down again. Now Samuel did not yet know the Lord, neither was the word of the Lord yet revealed to him. And the Lord called Samuel again the third time. And he arose and went to Eli, and said, here am I; for thou didst call me. And Eli perceived that the Lord had called the child. Therefore, Eli said unto Samuel, Go, lie down; and it shall be, if he calls thee, that thou shalt say, Speak Lord; for thy servant heareth. So, Samuel went and lay down in his place. And the Lord came, and stood, and called as at other times, Samuel, Samuel. Then Samuel answered, speak; for thy servant heareth.

Letting his Bible drop to his lap as he laid back in his chair and closed his heavy eyes, Tom suddenly heard audibly a quiet, compelling voice say, "Tom, are you listening?"

Tom's eyes shot open, and he was so startled that his Bible fell to the floor. He said nothing, supposing that he may have dozed off and was dreaming. But he had not been dreaming.

"Tom?" the deep, quiet, and reassuring voice came again.

"Yes," replied Tom in a terrified whisper.

"Do you want to hear me when I call and talk with me in the cool of the morning like my servant Enoch?"

"Yes," Tom whispered again.

"Then come to my holy mountain as a clean vessel," the voice said.

"What does that mean?" Tom asked in a louder voice, but the room was silent. Tom absentmindedly reached for his cup of coffee, and then stopped, placing it back upon the side table by his chair.

If that experience were not disquieting enough, the very next Saturday morning something strange and awe-inspiring happened as Reverend Dykes began to preach, walking down the center aisle while opening his Bible.

"The word today," Reverend Dykes said in a loud voice, "comes from the Book of Isaiah, Chapter Sixty-Six, Verse 20 – read along with me People of God:

> *And they shall bring all your brethren for an offering unto the Lord out of all nations upon horses, and in chariots, and in litters, and upon mules, and upon swift beasts, to my holy mountain Jerusalem, saith the Lord, as the children of Israel bring an offering in a clean vessel into the house of the Lord.*

"No! No!" a solitary voice rang out in the congregation.

Reverend Dykes stopped and turned his head to look at Tom Schmidt standing in the middle of a row of folding chairs near him. Most of the people in the congregation turned and looked as well.

"It can't be!" shouted Tom. "From the very lips of God, it can't be! This is not a coincidence! I have never read this passage before!"

Tom struggled over the legs of seated people in metal folding chairs until he reached the side aisle, and he turned running to the back of the church and out one of the huge doors. Gloria Singleton rose and followed behind him. Outside, Gloria found Tom leaning against the side of the barn over his bent arm, weeping.

"Tom," asked Gloria, "What's wrong? You'll freeze to death out here without your coat."

"It's God," said Tom with a heaving chest. "He talks to us."

"Of course, he does," said Gloria.

From that moment on Tom determined to first discover what a "clean vessel" was and then to become it so that he could talk to God as the voice had promised. Tom felt foremost that a clean vessel was probably a human body free of what could reasonably be classified as "pollutants". He completely gave up drinking coffee and all alcohol, but inasmuch as he could not hear the voice of God when he locked himself into his home office for morning prayer, he concluded that he was far from clean. He stopped eating any type of meat which his study of the Book of Deuteronomy revealed was scripturally unclean, despite Sueann's consternation one Sunday when she cooked her specialty, German pork roast and sauerkraut. Then Tom gave up meat altogether. Then he abandoned dairy products and eggs. And then yellow colored vegetables. But still there was no voice when he prayed in the mornings. It was as if the God had tantalized him with a burden, or test, and then had not appeared as promised regardless of how hard he had worked to make himself Biblically and spiritually a clean vessel.

Finally, it occurred to Tom to wash his hands carefully before he prayed by lifting up ostensibly "holy hands" as the Apostle Paul had written, even to the point of opening and closing the door of his home office with a Kleenex to avoid contamination. He at long last achieved his goal.

"Well done, Tom," the deep, soothing, and beautiful voice had said when Tom had prayed for God to "speak," because his "servant was listening."

Tom had wept for joy in his office as he held his hands skyward – as he had lifted "up holy hands in prayer" as had been directed long ago by the Apostle Paul. Then it all seemed so obvious. Like the Desert Fathers, Tom had – at God's direction – totally eliminated luxurious and polluting food and drink and made himself an empty vessel for God to speak.

It was addicting. Every morning Tom would speak with God in his office at home, and then the discussion would adjourn to his office at school where he would type the dictated text of his new book almost incessantly. At the university he never drank anything except water from the fountain, never chewed gum, and never ate lunch. In fact, Tom began to look upon all food rather suspiciously – even the white rice and cooked green cabbage he became nearly exclusively fond of eating for supper. The energy he received from speaking with God was far more exhilarating than the calories any food could offer. And then again – if there was even a slight chance that something he ate or drank, or even stray thoughts he might think, would end the voice of God . . . Tom shuddered at the thought. Never a particularly large man, Tom's weight dropped from 165 pounds to 140. Sueann begged him to see a doctor.

"No, Sueann," Tom would reply. "I know what I am doing. When my book is finished everything will return to normal." But Tom hoped it would never "return to normal". He did not want anything to ever "return to normal". He was ecstatic in a way he had never been before.

One December morning – as it turned out the one year anniversary of the Advent Awakening of the year before – Tom was busy at work typing in his office at school as a colleague came to the closed door and listened briefly to what he fancied was a vigorous conversation inside the little office.

"O.K., *now* I see what you are driving at," he could make out Tom saying.

He knocked lightly at the door.

"Come in," Tom said.

But to the colleague's surprise, when he opened the door Tom was the sole occupant of the office. The colleague chuckled.

"I'm sorry," he said. "I could have sworn I heard you talking with someone. Were you on the phone?"

"No," replied Tom with a smile, and then he added, "Oh maybe sort of. What can I do for you?"

"Ah," said the man. "Did you get the notice? This morning's department-wide meeting with Professor Hargrave about publishing deadlines?"

"Infernal meetings like this are doing their best to keep me from making the deadlines," Tom replied, "But I'll be there. Yes, I got the notice."

At the meeting that morning the history faculty was told by Professor Hargrave that a new policy had been instituted by the University Press for those faculty members wishing to utilize that outlet to publish textbooks, manuscripts or submit contributions to any of the twelve scholarly journals the University underwrote. The Professor announced contributors must first submit their works to their department heads for a preliminary content approval prior to sending them to the editorial staff of the press. In the case of department heads seeking to publish through the press, they would first have to submit their works to their respective college deans. Faculty members were not required to utilize this process, but publishing through the University Press automatically qualified as scholarly publication for tenure point advancement and side-stepped the necessity of peer review at the College of Liberal Arts level. In a poll taken by Professor Hargrave, Tom was one of the five hands held up signifying an intent by instructors, and full and associate professors, to utilize the University Press to publish their works in progress.

The first Saturday after the New Year, during the time of the service at the Church in the Fields set aside for prophecy, Tom got up from his seat by Gloria and went to stand in line at the front of the church. After a brief whispered discussion with Reverend Dykes, the pastor remarked, "Praise God, Brother Tom – tell that prophecy to the people!"

When his turn came Tom took the microphone, held up his copy of the King James Version of the Bible, and said, "Thus says the Lord your God, 'Beloved, I am the Truth and the Light. There is no other God than me. Yea further, there is no rule or law or code except my words. This Holy Book indeed contains my words. But also, my words are my words. Obey them all.' "

When the time for announcements came, Elder Cecile Gates took the microphone from off its stand and said, "As probably most of you know, next week is Iowa Solidarity for Life Week and it ends on Saturday with a large prayer service and rally in Des Moines where churches from all over Central Iowa will meet together to pray for the unborn and to picket the Lincoln Center abortion clinic on Lincoln Center Way in Des Moines.

Most of the Elders of the Church and the pastor have prayed over this, and we have reached a unanimous decision that we should not hold worship services next Sabbath here, in order to encourage all of us as is possible to go on one of the buses to Des Moines and pray and demonstrate for the unborn."

"Because of the size of the sign-up sheet," Gates continued, "we are leasing two buses to supplement our church bus, so there should be plenty of room for everybody who has either already signed up or decides this week to go. We will leave the church here promptly at 7 a.m. I mean promptly too, because we are intending to be on time for the big rally and prayer meeting at the Jesus Fellowship Community Tabernacle to be followed by the march to the clinic. If any of you aren't familiar with Pastor Green's church and will be driving in a private car, it's on I-101 right downtown off the High Street Exit toward the East. If you get to rubbernecking downtown and you see the West Street Exit to the left there you've gone too far, and you need to turn back and get off at High Street coming back south. No lunch will be provided. Within a couple of blocks of the clinic there is a Mr. Quickie and a Sven's Smorgasbord. Now, when we were up there last year picketing, both of these outfits were open, but we are told that there are going to be so many people there this time the police may very well order businesses along the parade route closed – so bring a lunch if you are in doubt or have special needs, even if you are a Quickie Burger fan. Mothers, there will be no nursery nor child-care facilities whatsoever. Pastor Green said they thought about it, but it was just logistically too big a mess to line up that many sitters. The march will be about nine blocks, so bear that in mind for the little ones if you bring them. We can accommodate a bunch of strollers in the leased buses' luggage compartments. We will not be getting arrested. That is not our cup of tea. I think it's fair to say that others will, but Pastor Dykes wants us there only for prayer support and the march – as for a sit-in or things of that nature we are out of our territory in Des Moines, and we have been advised by Brother Clifton, our lawyer, that it would be best to let the locals do what they need to do if anyone is going to be arrested. We want to all be back on the bus as a group when we're ready to go and be back in Madisonville by five. If you have any questions, ask either me or Elder Dave over yonder at the coffee pot."

At the coffee hour following the service, Gloria Singleton asked Tom, "Are you going on Saturday?"

"I might very well go," replied Tom. "It might be interesting."

"Tom," said Gloria sipping her coffee, "What did that prophesy you gave mean? The part about 'my words are my words'?"

"I don't know," answered Tom. "I don't know what God means sometimes."

Chapter Ten

At 6:30 in the morning the next Saturday Tom took a last gulp of milk from his glass and put a hand-written note under the rooster magnet on the refrigerator in his darkened kitchen. It read:

Sue – had to go in early today to work on my manuscript. Be back in time for supper – 5:30ish. Love, Tom

During the bus trip to Des Moines that morning everyone was animated and cheerful. Reverend Dykes and two of the music ministers from the Church were on Tom's bus, and the musicians lead the passengers in Jesus songs during the entire ride to the outskirts of the city. Reverend Dykes was dressed in a suit. As they began to pass the westernmost downtown exits, Reverend Dykes stood up in the aisle in the front part of the bus.

"O.K., folks, this is the drill," Reverend Dykes said. "We are only going to be prayer warriors and Godly support on this trip – meaning we want everybody in our group to try and stay out of police trouble as far as possible. If the demons of death infect the cops and they go wild we'll just have to do what we have to do, but I can tell you – I was arrested three years ago with the Minneapolis Loving for Life Group and it wasn't a whole lot of fun spending the night on a cold bench in central lock-up and showing up for jail call the next morning in a prison jump suit and flip-flops without socks. Stay together and keep your eyes on either me or one of the Elders in our group. You mothers with children in strollers – stay away from the Daughters of Deborah Group. This is a group of Roman Catholic women who Brother Green tells me are bringing their children to the clinic and after the initial sit-in and lockdown, and they are planning to stroll their kids right past the police lines and sit down with the first group – more or less daring the police to arrest them with the kids. I don't think it's much of a bluff, myself. You get to talking with the Catholic mothers and you pass the police line – you're going to go jail, pure and simple, and we're going to have to fetch your kids from Child Protection later on this afternoon."

"After the prayer meeting, we are going to march to the clinic, and then we are going to sing. Our own music ministers will lead us. The clinic has its own private guards to escort the women coming in. They don't carry weapons, but the City and State Police will be there in force. If the police get rough in the slightest way – that means grabbing, pushing, or dragging people on the street side of the protest line – we are all leaving, then and there. Pastor Green knows that – we've talked together, and he understands. Our church is not going to get caught up in rough shenanigans, and some of these people even on the Godly side of the protest line can irritate the heck out of the police."

For blocks on the approach to the Jesus Fellowship Community Tabernacle, parked cars lined the main thoroughfare and on every side street. Both parked and patrolling black and white Des Moines City Police squad cars and motorcycles were out in force, and most of the side streets adjacent to High Street had been barricaded by the police preparatory to the march. People lined the sidewalks of High Street, some carrying posters or crosses, and walked in both directions. The huge parking lot of the Jesus Fellowship Community Tabernacle was completely filled with the entrance gate blocked by two men. After a brief discussion with the driver of the first bus in the Church's convoy, the men backed up and waved the three vehicles through the gate.

As the line of buses drove through the parking lot toward the Church's main entrance, Tom could see out of the window at his seat that the circular shaped Tabernacle was huge and resembled a domed athletic arena more than a traditional church building. Adjacent to the entrance two large panel trucks were stationed, and atop one of the trucks several people stood as a television camera on a tripod panned the crowd milling in the parking lot and migrating toward the building's entrance. On one truck "KXTV Des Moines" was written, and on the other a sign proclaimed that the unit was "The Mobile Watchdog of KLLX Davenport."

Inside the Tabernacle Tom was flabbergasted at the seating capacity and size of the building. He thought that there was arguably space for ten thousand worshipers, and the interior was larger than the largest cathedral he had visited on his trip to Italy and Greece in graduate school. On an elevated platform close to the stage and podium down in front, two more television cameras were set up – probably a part of the church's own equipment – and fifty or more royal blue robed choir members were standing in three tiered rows to the rear of the stage. In what appeared to be an orchestra pit a significantly sized band with all types of instruments was assembled. Beside the podium on stage were two rows of folding chairs upon which were assembled a group of men in suits, which congregation Reverend Dykes proceeded to join in due course and take his place.

After the Church in the Fields group had made its way to a vast reserved seating area to the left behind the media platform, the band began to play a lively Jesus tune, and the choir began to clap their hands and sway with the music. Suddenly three large screens – one over the choir and one each to the right and left of the stage lit up with color televised images of the robed choir leader and part of the choir beginning to sing. White lettering superimposed over the picture of the choir on the screen flashed the words:

Innocents! Innocents! The Lord's innocents be saved!
Innocents! Innocents! The Lord's innocents be saved!

The growing congregation began to clap and sing along with the choir, and the chorus was sung two more times.

Innocents! Innocents! The Lord's innocents be saved!
Innocents! Innocents! The Lord's innocents be saved!

Then an attractive young female soloist with a hand-held microphone walked out onto the stage and over to the choir leader, singing. Her silver lamé ankle length dress shimmered in the overhead stage lights that panned the podium area back and forth.

Lord, you are the answer to all strife,
You are the reason for my life,
You are the newborn baby's cry
You wipe the tear from every eye.

"Innocents! Innocents! The Lord's innocents be saved!" echoed the hand clapping thousands that filled the auditorium. "Innocents! Innocents! The Lord's innocents be saved!"

Within thirty minutes time the Tabernacle had been filled, seemingly to capacity, and everyone was on his and her feet shouting, singing, and raising their hands. Eventually the music slowed, and the choir's collective voice lowered into a soft humming of sorts. On to the stage walked a smartly dressed middle-aged man with a handheld microphone.

"Let's just enter into prayer for a moment," he said arriving at the podium. "A moment of worship. Lord Jesus. Jehovah Jireh."

"Lord, you are so good to me," the man began to sing. "So good, so good, so good to me."

As the choir continued to hum, the leader said, "we are here today – on this glorious day – to both celebrate the goodness of the Lord and to beseech the Lord. To pray and beg and plead with the Lord that his unbelievable goodness and mercy be extended to the sweet little innocents scheduled to be executed today at the single most profitable and successful killing center in the State of Iowa. This death camp – this abortuary – run by a demented and demonic pitiful excuse for a physician has actually bragged to its investors and stockholders that it *averaged* twelve executions of little babies every weekday and Saturday last year. Can you imagine that? Can you imagine *bragging* about that shame and outrage to a group of Satan's minions who make their shameful livings off of the blood of little babies? I can't. Oh Jesus in Heaven, I can't! I swear by the holy blood of Jesus that were it not for the supernatural strength of the Holy Spirit I could not stand at this podium and even speak of such outrages to God and man. Oh Jesus, Oh Jesus, Oh Jesus give me the strength to say what must be said and to do what must be done to defend your little babies."

The leader, who Tom guessed was Reverend Green, paused for a moment to weep, hiding his face in his free hand. Then he reached into his breast coat pocket to extract a handkerchief and wiped his eyes. Putting away the handkerchief, he reached into his inside coat pocket and extracted what looked to be a multi-page document, flipping it to its unfolded state with a snap of his wrist and hand.

"Last night," he continued, "as I knelt in prayer in my living room for the unborn children of this city and state, a knock came on my door. It was the Sheriff of Polk County and two of his deputies."

"They handed me this," the man said holding up the paper, "and they explained to me that the owners of the Lincoln Center abortuary had obtained an injunction against me prohibiting me or any member of my church from approaching closer than one hundred yards to the killing center today. They apologized, and they said they were sorry but if I or any of my brothers or sisters in this church violated the injunction, they would be forced to arrest us. It was the injunction, you see. Well, I told the officers that it was *I* who should apologize. It was *I* who was sorry and sorry for them, because it looked as if *they* would be the ones who would be arrested today – their hearts and their tears and their consciousnesses and indeed their very souls would be arrested as they dragged away Christian brothers and sisters to jail. You see, I already had an *injunction* which had been served on me before the Sheriff ever rang my doorbell. The *Lord God Almighty* spoke to me, and I had an injunction from God himself. The Lord God Jehovah had already *enjoined* me to save the unborn – and Beloved, that is an order from the heavenly court that one dare not disobey, even on pain of imprisonment, even on pain – dare I say it – of death."

"Well," said the preacher, "do you wanted to know what happened *then* last night?"

"Yes! Praise God!" people shouted from the filled auditorium.

"We prayed together – that's what we did Praise God!" said the man. "I invited those officers – two men and one woman – into my living room and we prayed together for them, for their families, and for the unborn. Beloved, don't you see what this scourge of abortion is doing to us as a country and a state and a city? A blind man could see it! At some point good and lawful and Godly men of all stations in life – even our elected officials – must say No! Enough! I am not going to support wickedness!"

"Well," he continued, "let me ask you this. Do you know what's going to happen to me *today*?"

Many people in the huge auditorium laughed.

"Well *today*," said the speaker, "I'm going to pray for the Sheriff *again*, only this time it's probably going to be from jail." The man let the legal paper flutter to the stage floor. Scattered people in the auditorium laughed or said "amen!"

"Because," he said pointing, "Right now I am going to walk down those stairs over there, and I am going to walk out of those glass doors back there, and I am going to walk down the street to the Lincoln Center abortuary and I am going to hand a little tract to any woman who tries to keep an appointment with death today – I don't care how big and menacing her security guard escort is – until they arrest me, and when I am sitting on a bench in my jail cell tonight I am going to pray for those deluded young women and their poor, poor babies. If any of you would like to join me, I have asked that a few additional tracts about the sanctity of life be made available. We have about fifteen thousand of them sitting in three big boxes up there by the doors. You can pick up a handful and follow me down the street. Hallelujah!"

The band began to play a rousing song as the words flashed on the screens, and the choir and congregation began to sing and rhythmically clap their hands. The speaker raised one hand above his head and marched down the stage steps up the center aisle and out the double glass doors of the auditorium, followed by the two dozen or so men in suits who had sat behind him on stage – including Reverend Dykes.

Outside of the Tabernacle Tom found the scene both chaotic and colorful. People of all ages – from those on crutches to little ones in strollers – walked, rolled, hobbled, talked, sang, and shouted as they moved down High Street and under the Interstate 101 overpass in a large but generally orderly jumble. Some carried signs or posters. Many carried crosses of all descriptions on poles. Police sirens blared in the distance, and police officers of all description and types of uniforms lined the streets or walked along side of the crowds. That night on the KLLX Davenport six o'clock news a Des Moines Police spokeswoman would estimate the marchers at about 8,000, but on the KXTV Des Moines nightly news after the

Hawkeyes game, Mayor Rodney Stoltz put the number of marchers closer to 12,000.

A few blocks past the I-101 underpass, at a place where High Street merges into Lincoln Center Way, Tom began to hear a second chorus of song singing coming from the right up Lincoln. Soon he could make out the words clearly:

> *All hail the power of Jesus' name*
> *Let angels prostrate fall*
> *Bring forth the royal diadem*
> *And crown him Lord of all.*
> *Bring forth the royal dia – aha – dem*
> *And crown him Lord of all.*

To Tom's amazement a *second* large group of marchers was proceeding down Lincoln Center Way and beginning to merge into and walk with the Tabernacle group. Leading the Lincoln Center Way marchers was a group of about thirty men, two of whom were carrying a blue and yellow marching banner on a long pole announcing "Knights of Columbus, King of Jerusalem Council 9887." Behind the men there were seven or eight black-clad priests with white round Roman collars showing beneath their jackets. Following the priests was a hodgepodge of singing marchers and many children, some carrying crucifixes or rosaries – or both. Two teenagers moving along with the marchers were handing out fliers printed on green paper to onlookers lining the parade route. Then Tom saw a banner proclaiming "The Prophetic Daughters of Deborah." From all appearances, the banner identified the group of mothers Reverend Dykes had warned the women on the bus about, and indeed behind the banner carrier came fifteen- or twenty-women pushing strollers, some with older children on foot in tow as well.

As the marchers neared the Lincoln Center Family Clinic a line of police officers, perhaps a hundred in number, could be seen spread out in a line on the Clinic side of the street on the sidewalk. The marchers swarmed down the street and all along the police line down to the street's intersection with Wilke Way. One officer with multiple stripes on his sleeve walked to and fro all up and down the street between the block-long lines of protestors and officers.

At first the demonstration appeared to Tom to be totally chaotic and unorganized. The television crews had re-located to positions across the street from the clinic, and newspaper photographers wandered through the crowds snapping pictures.

"Sinners!" a man with a large crucifix standing near Tom shouted. "You whores of Babylon! Witches! Murderers! You are going to a murderer's everlasting death in hell!"

"Killers!" a woman standing in front of Tom screamed. She was wearing a sweatshirt with a picture of a newborn on the front and "Protect the Unborn" printed on the back. Three scapulars, or small Roman Catholic green and white prayer cloths suspended by strings, hung around her neck outside of her sweatshirt, and she held on to the hand of a child who looked to be about seven years old.

Just then a young man – possibly in his early twenties – ran out from the crowd carrying what looked like two gallon cans of red paint, one in each hand. At least Tom could see a Benjamin Moore Paint label on one of them. He stopped abreast of the abortion clinic's driveway about ten feet from the nearest police officer and proceeded to pour the red substance – one can after the other – into the street.

"Oh, Mother of God!" Tom heard a voice say, and he turned to see two Roman Catholic priests standing behind him. "What's that idiot doing?" the voice continued.

"You know," said the other priest to his colleague, "the Bishop has considerable influence with the Police Commissioner – he's even Catholic – but not when these psychos act like this."

Turning back around, Tom saw the two cans sitting at the man's feet in a pool of what was probably red paint – who knew for sure. The man had produced a folded sheet of white paper from his pocket, and had turned to the line of protestors, unfolding the document.

"A poem on the sacredness of life and the spilling of blood!" the man read in a loud voice to the crowd.

Suddenly three police officers rapidly came forward from behind the street poet, and two of them simultaneously grabbed the man by the shoulders, twisting his arms behind him with one of the captured hands still clutching the paper. However, the third officer was somehow knocked off balance in the arm-twisting struggle and suddenly slipped. Both of his feet flew out from beneath him, and he landed in the pool of red goo.

"Oh Jesus!" the first priest behind Tom said disgustedly. "It just gets worse."

As the two standing officers held the man and affixed a black plastic flex cuff around his wrists behind his back, the fallen officer struggled to his feet. He was a crimson-colored mess.

"God damn it!" Tom heard the officer exclaim to his colleagues. "A twenty-eight-dollar pair of pants and my best long sleeve uniform shirt!"

Tom's attention was suddenly drawn to the far end of the street near the intersection with Wilke Way. He turned his head to see a group of about fifty people – lead by Pastor Green – running behind the police line at full speed over the lawn of the clinic and up to the front double glass doors. The protestors had apparently seized upon the confusion created by the paint-pouring street poet to do an "around end" maneuver at the far end of the police line and rush the clinic's entrance from the side.

"Good move!" said one of the priests behind Tom. "Hayden Fry could have used that guy out in front in the Holiday Bowl. He's as fast as Cook." The other priest laughed.

The protestors scooted together in three rough lines across the front door of the clinic, and linked arms. They began singing, and soon several thousand protestors in the street, on the north sidewalk, and even between the buildings on the north side of the street began singing in unison.

Were you there when they crucified my Lord?
Were you there when they crucified my Lord?
Ohhhh, sometimes it makes me tremble, tremble, tremble.
Were you there when they crucified my Lord?

The vanguard of the entrenched attackers at the clinic's doors had not even got to the verse of the hymn asking whether the listener had been there when "he rose up from the grave" before a black and white painted police bus had made its way through the crowds on the street to the clinic and uniformed officers had begun escorting the barricaders in handcuffs to the vehicle. Most of the protestors walked and cooperated with their arrests, but several refused to walk and had to be carried to the open back door of the bus and ignominiously dumped in.

Although successive waves of protestor rushes to the clinic doors may have been planned for that afternoon, actually only one more succeeded before the Church in the Fields gathered its group together and walked back to the Tabernacle's parking lot to the buses. That happened when the suit-clad group of men who had sat with Pastor Green and Reverend Dykes on stage that morning assembled as if on cue in front of the police line about an hour after the first group of door barricaders had been taken away in the police bus. After convening in a huddled group, the men began to pray and weep and wail with hands raised in a considerable din that attracted the attention of protestors and the police alike.

Carefully side-stepping the very nasty puddle of red with bus tracks traced through it, the men spread out in two lines, and then simultaneously fell upon their faces – in their dress suits no less – upon the tarmac of the street. Lying prostrate they continued their weeping and wailing in loud voices.

"Careful," the police officer in charge called out. "Watch the flanks!"

Suddenly, from behind Tom he heard a voice of one of the priests who had been standing next to him for some time.

"Oh Rod!" the priest called out in a loud voice. "Rodney Riley!"

One of the uniformed officers just to the west of the red paint spill suddenly looked up in the direction of the Tom and the two priests.

"I didn't know you were here!" The priest behind Tom yelled.

The officer said something inaudible to the priest.

"I can't hear you!" yelled the priest. "What?"

The officer moved to the right near the center of the paint spill and cupped his hands to his mouth to say something over the noise of the prostrate clerics' shouting and moaning. Just then a line of thirty-five to fifty protestors ran from the crowd through the prone ministers at full speed and on through the gap in the line created by Officer Rod Riley.

"God damn it!" the officer in charge shouted – to no one in particular

– as he looked around to see the second wave of protestors seated and huddled arm in arm at the clinic's door.

"You sly bastard," Tom heard one of the priests behind him say to the other. "That was very good, a veritable quarterback sneak. Where did you learn that one?"

"Notre Dame, '68 – red shirted for one year, then they gave me the boot," his friend said. After a pause, he continued, "Oh don't give me that look – we have to work with the heretics every so often or they'll claim we're not Christians."

On his walk back to the Tabernacle with the Church in the Fields group, a stranger walked up to Tom with a jar containing something floating in liquid.

"What's that?" Tom asked.

"What do you think that is?" the man responded.

"That's frightening," said Tom.

"We live in frightening times, my brother," the man had responded.

The atmosphere in Tom's bus on the way back to Madisonville that afternoon was not festive.

"Oh Lord," one of the women prayed out loud, "I pray for the little babies that we were not able to save today. Forgive us for the killings we were not able to prevent."

Yet, in a way, Tom was confused. For sure the day had been exhilarating, and in terms of sheer numbers of people even more than the Iowa State Vietnam War protests in the '70s he had witnessed. But in truth and in fact, he had not seen even one woman go into the clinic that day – or try to. There had been a lot of talk about private security guards and the wicked abortionist. But he had not seen anyone go into or leave the clinic in the hours he had stood, sang, and prayed in Lincoln Center Way. The Prophetic Daughters of Deborah had not rushed forward with their children in arms and dared the police to arrest them. How much of the anti-abortion movement was television cameras, crowds, and public displays – and how much of it was something that – as a man – he could not even fathom in the depths of his heart or conceivably understand the issues presented to the mind of a terrified young woman? Tom did not know. He would ask God tomorrow morning during his prayer time.

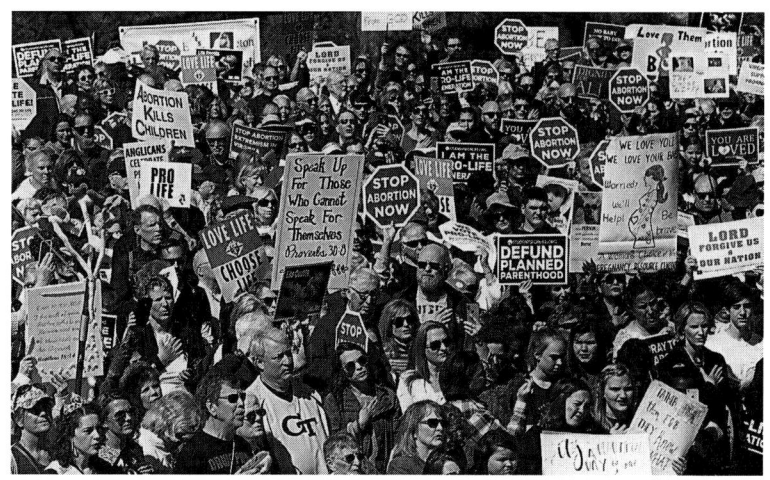

Chapter Eleven

"Tom, can you come over right away?" Reverend Dykes' voice came over the phone one Wednesday afternoon in February.

"I don't know," Tom had said. "I'm busy working on my new book, and I have office hours for the students later on."

"Well, can you put a note on the door or get someone else to do that this afternoon?" Reverend Dykes asked. "It's the Miller couple, you know the new ones from Davenport? There's serious trouble. I need you and a couple other trusted Elders of the church to help. We'll meet at the church as soon as you can get here. Bring a cross if you have one."

With the foreboding and puzzling introduction turning over in his mind, Tom pulled the Celtic cross off of the office wall, stuffed it into his jacket pocket, and hurriedly drove out to the Church in the Fields. In the parking lot were four other cars, and Reverend Dykes was standing in a group of three other men – all Elders – who Tom recognized. After greetings they all climbed into Elder Dave Woods' Suburban and rode together on a long ride to the couple's home south of the Little Otoe River.

"What's up?" Tom asked on the ride. It seemed to him that all of the other men were very much more up to speed on what was happening than was he.

"Let's just see what is happening when we get there, Brother Tom," replied Reverend Dykes.

When the group of men was admitted to the house by Mr. Miller, a bizarre scene presented itself. Mr. Miller, a man of about twenty-five, was naked to the waist and smeared here and there with blood, which may have come primarily from his right hand that was greatly injured by the looks of it. The small two-bedroom house was in total shambles with seemingly everything overturned, and the contents of shelves and drawers scattered about the floor. The faucet and one of the control knobs on the kitchen sink were gone, and water was spraying straight up into the air like a fountain and falling back down into the sink. A brick post about ten inches in diameter separating the dining-living area from the kitchen had been shattered in the middle and was only hanging together by metal rebar wire in the middle of the post.

"I got this," Mr. Miller said holding up his mangled hand, "when I hit the post."

Tom wondered to himself, "how many times?"

Mrs. Miller herself was the strangest aspect of the home, though. She was perched on the top back of the living room couch in a squat position barefoot and in her nightgown. She grinned widely and stared at the group of men as sweat stuck her hair to her forehead.

"Ro sha, sha, ka ba, ra shema," Reverend Dykes said as he began to move towards the woman. He approached Mrs. Miller slowly and cautiously as he took a large silver metallic cross from his jacket pocket and held it out – not *to* her but *at* her. Mrs. Miller started to laugh hysterically.

"Ro sha, sha, ka ba, ra shema!" the Reverend repeated. "In Jesus' name come out of that woman!"

"You can't hurt me," Mrs. Miller sneered at Reverend Dykes as she laughed. Tom thought there was undeniably a wild and irrational look in her eye, but the same could have easily been said of Mr. Miller.

"She did it. She did it," Mr. Miller said haltingly as he broke into tears. "In my own bed – in my own bed, Pastor Dykes. She had sex with my best friend in my own bed! Oh, this wasn't the only time. Two years ago, she said it would never happen again. She said she would never do that again – but she did. IN MY OWN BED! In my own bed. In my own bed . . ."

Mr. Miller was hysterical and beside himself. On her perch Mrs. Miller was giggling continually. Tom shuddered and pulled the Celtic cross from his pocket if for no other reason than to reassure himself. The woman seemed to have a certifiably demonic grin on her face. Just then the door burst open and a larger delegation of men and women from the Church in the Fields came into the wasted living room. Apparently, someone or multiple persons had put out the call for the "prayer line" of volunteers to come over and help out.

"You poor child!" one of the women exclaimed, as she took off her coat and placed it around Mrs. Miller's shoulders. Two other women helped Mrs. Miller down from her perch on the couch, and before too many minutes had elapsed the newly formed women's delegation had located Mrs. Miller's house slippers, swept Mrs. Miller out of the house, and taken her away in one of the cars.

"In my own bed!" Mr. Miller was explaining to two of the newly arrived men, one of who had braved the blood and sweat and a terrible odor coming from Mr. Miller to place his arm around the young man.

"He needs a doctor," one of the Elders said. "His hand has stopped bleeding, but he still needs a doctor. I think he needs stitches."

One of the men found a dirty men's shirt on the bedroom floor and helped Mr. Miller on with it, and Mr. Miller was taken away to the emergency room. The Elders and Reverend Dykes were left to lock up. One of the men knelt in the wet brick debris on the kitchen floor, reaching under the sink to find a cut-off valve for the water.

Addressing no one in particular, Reverend Dykes said, "You know, I try and not see a demon behind every bush. In this business if you do that pretty soon all you'll be doing is fighting demons. But that little witch was demon-possessed. I'd stake my soul on it."

In the next two weeks Mr. Miller showed up faithfully on Saturday at the Church in the Fields with his bandaged right hand in a sling. He came to the front of the church and asked for healing prayers during the general invitation made by Reverend Dykes. On the third week, to Tom Schmidt's utter amazement Mr. Miller's former "best friend" walked into the church service just as Mr. Miller was yet again receiving prayers for healing by Reverend Dykes at the front of the congregation. In tears, the friend – also a young man in his early twenties – walked to the front of the congregation and fell to his knees before an equally astonished Reverend Dykes and Mr. Miller. In a loud voice the former friend tearfully asked for Mr. Miller's and God's forgiveness while on his knees, and Mr. Miller himself fell to his knees and hugged the man with his left, uninjured, arm. The congregation broke into shouts of "Praise God," and the music ministers returned to their instruments and began playing.

Lord, you are so good
You are so very good to me.

At the coffee hour following the service, Gloria Singleton filled Tom in on some of the details of the entire Miller incident that Tom had not been aware of. Several women of the church had befriended Mrs. Miller, and she was now living at a church member's house. A collection was quietly being taken up so that Mrs. Miller could re-establish herself and enroll at the business college in town. Reverend Dykes apparently would have nothing to do with the collection and had refused to announce it in church. The church was slowly being divided into two cliques, a pro-Mr. Miller clique and a "Mr. Miller is nothing more than a wife beater" pro-Mrs. Miller clique.

"There's something *really* goofy about this whole drama," Gloria said sipping her coffee.

The next week Gloria's impression was apparently confirmed when, at the coffee hour, Gloria revealed to Tom that the woman with whom Mrs. Miller had been living reported both Mr. and Mrs. Miller were gone. They were said to have reconciled and gone back to Davenport.

Chapter Twelve

After a consuming winter and spring of intense writing, Tom submitted a first draft of "*Post-Modern Trends in Christian History*" to Professor Hargrave for review. Although the professor promised to be back in touch with Tom on his impressions of the book in a couple of weeks, it was not until mid-April that Tom got a call one day from Professor Hargrave wondering if Tom could come down the hall and step into his office for a few moments, right away.

"Sit down, Tom," the professor said in a business-like manner when Tom entered his office. "Why don't you close the door."

"Tom," the professor continued as Tom took a seat facing the desk, "I must confess at the outset that I only got a chance to sit down with your book's draft for the first time last night at home. I spent a few hours with it last night and some more time with it this morning."

"Yes," said Tom with a broad smile.

"Tom," said the professor, "I don't want to be disrespectful in the least – but I must ask you if your submission of this manuscript was intended to be serious."

"Meaning what, Professor Hargrave?" Tom asked.

"Well," replied the professor, "there are over three hundred type written pages here – that must be a hundred thousand words . . ."

"A hundred fourteen thousand words," interrupted Tom.

"My point is," said the professor, "for a joke it is a bizarrely elaborate and very time-consuming one."

"What do you mean a joke?" asked Tom. "This is a serious work – one I think of unprecedented importance."

Tom's facial expression looked concerned and expressed genuine confusion. The professor's face likewise exhibited concern.

"Tom, let me approach it this way," said the professor. "As an ostensible scholar and the head of this department I enjoyed reading your first book comparing the Byzantine expression of orthodoxy to the Counter Reformation very much. I've got it over there on one of my shelves. But, Tom, that was a genuine work of scholarship. You documented your references well. I recall you had several hundred footnotes and an extensive bibliography. You have proved your ability. However, if we were to submit this manuscript to the University Press editorial board – you, me and our department would be the laughingstock of the University."

"That's not just a little bit disheartening," replied Tom. "I can't believe you are saying that. This book is unprecedented. This book is groundbreaking. Can you imagine in print for the first time the very words of . . . ?"

Tom stopped speaking suddenly and stared at the ceiling, biting his lip and overcome with some kind of emotion Professor Hargrave could not discern was anger or disappointment, or both.

"Tom," the professor asked sincerely, "are you all right?"

"No," said Tom. "I'm not all right. Give me the book back, and I'll get it published off campus. There will be many publishing houses that will want to publish this. This book is an answer to the world's cry for help."

"I'm sorry," said Professor Hargrave handing the manuscript over the desk to Tom.

"You'll see. You'll see," said Tom taking the manuscript and rising. "I'll make the deadline." Tom disappeared through the door, stomped across the department secretary's office, and disappeared down the hallway.

"What's with him?" Charlotte Middlebury, the secretary, asked, sticking her head into the professor's office.

"Insanity," said Professor Hargrave quite seriously. "Tom Schmidt is as crazy as a loon."

However, as dismissive as Professor Hargrave's words to Charlotte may have sounded out loud, he was deeply troubled about both what he had read in Tom's manuscript and in Tom's reaction in the meeting with him. In fact, he was so troubled that at ten o'clock he asked Ray Timmermann to take his Medieval Apologetics class so that he could make a telephone call.

"Hello," answered Sueann Schmidt pleasantly into the telephone.

"Mrs. Schmidt," said the professor, "this is Brent Hargrave from Harvest Christian University."

"Yes, Professor Hargrave," Sueann replied. "How can I help you – is something wrong?"

"It's my great fear that there might be," said the professor. "Do you have a second to talk?"

"Yes, of course, professor," answered Sueann. "Is there something the matter with Tom? Is he all right?"

"Well, I'm not sure," the professor said haltingly, and then he quickly corrected himself, "no, that came out wrong – Tom's fine – I mean *physically* – nothing has happened – he just left my office a little while ago, and he's *physically* fine."

"Something's wrong, Professor Hargrave," Sueann replied with a concerned voice. "Please tell me what is the matter."

"Well, Mrs. Schmidt," he said, "You are aware of course that Tom has been working on a book to submit to the University Press for publishing?"

"Yes, of course," answered Sueann. "He's worked on it day and night for months. He said it was finished a month ago."

"Mrs. Schmidt," asked the professor, "have you read the book or has Tom read any of it to you?"

"No," said Sueann. "History is not my thing, and religious history is *really* not my thing. Why, is there something wrong with his book?"

"Mrs. Schmidt," the professor asked evasively, "has Tom been acting, well, less than himself lately, especially in the area of religion?"

There was total silence on the line.

After a few seconds Professor Hargrave spoke again, "Mrs. Schmidt, are you still there?"

"Yes," Sueann replied. As she spoke it became clear from her cracked voice that she was crying. "I'm still here – Tell me about Tom's book."

"It's a very unusual book, Mrs. Schmidt," the professor replied. "It's not traditional or scholarly in any sense of the word. It's more like a compilation of widely dissimilar fragments. Some of it is a kind of historical narrative, but there are also poems and what can be loosely described as accounts of dreams or visions. But its form is not what concerns me as much as what it purports to be. In the forward to the book Tom asserts that God, or *some* god, has dictated to him what to write down. He claims that his was just a stenographic role and that the light of this god – personified by the Sun – shined into him producing some kind of ecstasy and told him what to type. He claims no pride in authorship."

"Oh dear," Sueann said sniffing.

"It is so bizarre that at first I thought it was a joke," the professor continued. "I think I inadvertently insulted him. He took back the book in my office this morning and stomped out."

"Ah, Mrs. Schmidt," Professor Hargrave said. "The purpose of my call is actually two-fold. First, I wanted to assure myself that from the perspective of Tom's wife this comes as new information to you, and you are concerned in the same sense as I am. Is that correct?"

"Yes, professor, you are certainly correct about that," replied Sueann.

"Well, on the assumption that was a correct impression," said the professor, "the second purpose of my call was to suggest a possible consultation by Tom, or you and Tom, or even you alone with a professional counselor or psychologist-type in order to determine what the heck is going on. Communication between Tom and me has obviously broken down. At this point I don't know if Tom's book is just some type of academic protest or whether it stems from some kind of underlying dissatisfaction Tom has with the University. I hate to sound crass, and my first concern is for Tom of course, but this is a private Christian university and we have a multitude of hyper-sensitive parents that prick up their ears at the slightest sound of what they construe to be religious heresy. I shudder to think what the gossip mill will be saying if news of Tom's book gets out. It could really cause some trouble not only for Tom but for the department and the university."

"I think I get what you're saying," Sueann replied sadly. "I'll see what I can do."

"There is a good man in town named Newman Scott," said Professor Hargrave. "I don't want to be presumptuous in suggesting a person, but quite confidentially he helped me considerably with a little problem I was having with my youngest daughter two years ago. Not only is he competent, but he is a Christian and can be trusted. I have his number right here if you would like it."

Sueann asked for the number, more out of politeness than with a definite plan in mind because she utterly had no idea what to do. It took her awhile, through two loads of laundry and a reorganization of the boys' bedroom toy box, just to fully digest what the professor had told her. Finally, Sueann had to admit to herself, however painful that admission was, that she had been hiding the implications of Tom's behavior in recent months even from herself.

Tom *wasn't* all right. Nothing stuck out so obviously that Sueann could put her finger on a definite problem, but at the same time there were dozens of little things that she had noted and then dismissed in denial. These days Tom rarely came to bed before the wee hours of the morning, and then often tossed and turned with insomnia until he got up again and disappeared into his home office with the foyer door closed. He was a picky eater to the point of being ridiculous. In fact, Sueann rarely knew what he ate at all. He had not sat down to a meal with her and the boys for months. He had lost weight and refused to go to a doctor even though they had good health insurance through the university. Yet without sleeping and without eating, he seemed full of energy most of the time until he just seemed to collapse from a cumulative lack of rest and would sleep for ten or twelve hours. And he was secretive. Very secretive. If Tom didn't need counseling, Sueann thought, something else was going on, and it was going to wreck their home life if she didn't get to the bottom of it. It may have already affected Tom's job at the university.

"That son of a bitch!" Tom shouted that evening in the living room when Sueann told him about Professor Hargrave's call. "That jealous, backstabbing, academic son of a bitch! I'm glad I got my book back from him. He probably copied the thing and is plagiarizing the text as we speak. You did right in telling me about this."

"Tom?" Sueann said with an inquiring voice, "Are you all right? I mean do you feel all right? You haven't slept well in weeks."

"I've never felt better," said Tom enthusiastically, and in fact he looked to Sueann as if he really *was* energized.

"Tom," Sueann said, "Professor Hargrave told me a little about the book."

"Bastard!" Tom said. "He shouldn't have told anybody about the book. He's probably blabbing about it to everyone he knows right now."

"Wasn't that the point of the exercise?" Sueann asked. "I mean to get the book published through the University Press?"

"Published, yes," said Tom. "Printed, yes, but it has to be released at the right time. I really haven't been given the . . . I really haven't *decided* when it should be released to the public."

"Tom," Sueann said touching his right arm and looking into his eyes with a genuinely concerned expression on her face, "I want us to go to a counselor together. I'm worried about you. You don't eat. You don't sleep. Now there's trouble with the department chairman. Maybe you need to relax. Get a prescription for some sleeping pills or something – I don't know. I just know your behavior is not normal lately, and it's really beginning to affect our marriage."

"I've got a counselor, Sue," replied Tom. "I already have a counselor. The best one in the universe, and certainly the best one in Madisonville."

"And this counselor is?" asked Sueann incredulously.

"Well, I don't know about names that would make any sense to you," replied Tom. "Let's say I have the most enlightened counselor possible and leave it at that."

Sueann did leave it at that. In silence she fed and bathed the boys as Tom retreated to his home office, and in silence later she closed the door of the bedroom, turned off the light, got under the covers – and cried. At two in the morning she woke briefly as Tom got into bed. After forty-five minutes of tossing and turning Tom got up and disappeared out into the dark hallway, leaving the door to the bedroom open.

"Oh God," Sueann said to herself sobbing in a half-prayer. "Help us."

Chapter Thirteen

The next morning after Tom had left for work and the boys were organized, Sueann went into the home office off the foyer with a mission. She wanted to find Tom's book and see for herself what he had written. Rationalizing her initial alarm at Professor Hargrave's call, she thought to herself that maybe Tom was right, and the professor's criticism of the book was simply academic jealousy of some kind.

Beside the desk and propped up against it was Tom's old leather briefcase that he occasionally took to school. Seizing the case, Sueann unlatched the cover and looked inside not really expecting to find the book because of the lack of heft it provided. However, what she found utterly flabbergasted her in a way even the book at its worst might not have. Attached with a paperclip was a yellow University Mail eight by ten-inch envelope, a newspaper clipping, and a white sticky note. In handwriting the note read:

> *Tom – My friend Allyson who lives in Des Moines sent me this clipping. You're famous! Praise God!*
> *Love,*
> *Gloria*

The newspaper article had been taken from the Sunday *Des Moines Leader* and bore a date nearly four months earlier, discussing the abortion clinic protests in Des Moines. As if printed in bold letters, the words of the article "a contingent as far away as the Church in the Fields in Madisonville" caught Sueann's gaze nearly simultaneously and in competition with the picture accompanying the article. As the caption announced, there, standing with two priests with black shirts and collars was . . . was "Elder Tom Schmidt from Church in the Fields." *Her* Tom Schmidt.

In a twinkling, Sueann's concern for and even defense of her husband changed from compassion to rage, and she was beside herself in confusion and anger. She utterly now had no idea who she was married to or what kind of life he had been living outside of their suburban home. No wonder Tom didn't act like himself. He wasn't himself. He was someone else she no longer knew and certainly had no reason to trust.

Trying to compose herself, Sueann telephoned Sarah Jenkins next door and asked if the older woman would be kind enough to watch the boys while she ran an important errand. Sarah said "of course" – as she always did, and in two or three minutes the kindly neighbor was standing in the doorway as Sueann gave her a quick hug and hurriedly walked to her car with her purse and a clutched handful of papers.

"So, who's Gloria?" Sueann demanded in a loud voice as she threw the stack of papers with the newspaper article on Tom's desk at the university.

"Gloria? I mean Sueann. What are you doing here?" a startled Tom Schmidt answered looking up. "Come in. Shut the door."

"The hell with the door!" Sueann shouted. "Who's Gloria?"

"She's just a friend – an acquaintance from . . ." Tom stuttered.

"From what?" demanded Sueann interrupting. "From Church in the Fields? You promised me we won't go as a family to that place, so you – what – sneak off with Gloria Whoever to it when you think I'm not looking? And you're in Des Moines at some kind of rally with a couple of priests when you swear to me your working on your book?"

"I, I wanted to tell you, Sue – not about Gloria – she's just a friend from the university here. I swear that's all. But I wanted to tell you about the Church in the Fields. I guess I just didn't think you'd *understand*. That's all."

"The book!" Sueann demanded. "I want a copy of the book right now, and I'm not leaving without it. You know what I'm talking about."

Tom reached over to the left side of his desk and handed Sueann a clip-bound three-inch collection of white pages with a red press-board cover. Grabbing the book brusquely from his hand Sueann turned and stomped out of the open door and toward the parking lot exit. Two or three startled onlookers in the hallway who had emerged from their offices upon hearing the voices, suddenly looked up or turned around in a vain attempt to appear nonchalant.

After returning home, Sueann's first destination was the cupboard beside the refrigerator in the kitchen where she took out the bottle of red wine she had purchased for her and Tom's anniversary dinner – a bottle of wine, parenthetically, Tom had declined to share in as he had basically declined the roast beef dinner she had fixed, eating only the boiled potatoes and snap beans. At the time he had offered to open the wine and pour just her a glass in order to toast their health with his own glass of mineral water, but she had indignantly refused. Now, with the fear her marriage was crumbling before her very eyes, she thought it more than apropos to open the ill-fated bottle herself and pour a drink. Or two. Or possibly three depending how she felt.

Sitting on the divan in the den, she took a long drink of the wine, curled her feet under herself, and opened the book.

"Jesus!" She thought to herself as she flipped through the pages. "If anything, Professor Hargrave had soft-peddled the insanity of the thing." There was the introduction all right where Tom asserted that he was "but an instrument of the Uncreated Light and wrote only as directed by it." The chapters appeared to be organized loosely as a type of parallel to the Bible, beginning with "New Genesis" and ending with "The Apocalypse of Love." Just as Professor Hargrave had said, there were whole chapters that looked to be in a kind of poetic verse, while others were in prose organized into many sub-chapters. However, she did not think what she read was complete gibberish. In fact, as she sipped her wine – more slowly now – read excerpts and turned the pages some of the things she read seemed quite beautiful to her. The first partition of the book was labeled "The Timeless Testament." In the chapter "New Genesis" she read:

> *You are Creation's eyes, Creation's ears.*
> *You are Creation's tongue and heart and soul.*
> *You are the fruitful field, the wind, the stars.*
> *You are the rolling wave upon the shore.*
> *You each are Creation in celebration*
> *Of all that was and will be ever more.*

None has a true beginning birth, and none will die.
All are the ancient oak and rocky crag.
All are the rain that falls upon the earth,
And yet the moon that that lights the midnight sky.
Know this in starry ecstasy at night:
All is all in God's eternal sight.

Sueann was not sure what some of the things she read meant, but the words themselves at times sounded quite lovely and even moving. In "Never Exodus" she read:

There are those who mindlessly argue that Adam and Eve transgressed in the Garden of Eden, and that their union was cursed in original sin with hard toil for the man and painful childbirth for the woman. Do you not understand that the love union of two humans is the greatest gift and joy God has bestowed upon the human race? A love union is not a vehicle for difficult toil. It is not simply some mechanism whereby children can be conceived and born. An employment – the most casual and brief liaison – can accomplish these things. No, the love union of two humans is an eternal celebration. An act of completion. An act of acceptance of all that is. Fulfillment of being. An expression of the cosmic glue of celestial love that holds all of creation together. Adam and Eve did not sin in their mutual love, nor even in their desire to give immortality to their beloved by exchanging the forbidden fruit from the Tree of Life. They loved. They risked all for love. Would you not risk all for true and complete love? What is death to one who lives without love?

In the chapter "Song of Celestial Love" she read:

I've seen you in a dozen, dozen forms:
The soaring gull and flying fish at sea,
The caterpillar on the morning vine,

The dragon fly which often visits me.
Here is the oleander in bright bloom,
And flowers' wild arrayed in glory seen.
But most of all the sun beams, now under,
Now through, the clouds – seem visitations true
As golden life-lines leading back to you.

Flipping over to the partition of the book entitled "The Newer Testament", Sueann read in the chapter "Everyone Every Time":

Why argue, quarrel, persecute and even kill one another over the supposed divinity of Jesus of Nazareth? Rather, listen to his words:

As Sueann turned the pages she saw where the words "Love your neighbor" in succession in the middle of the page was the only thing written for the fifteen following pages until the end of the chapter.

Closing the book carefully, Sueann laid it beside her on the divan, and slowly sipped her wine. A tear, then two, and then a flood of silent tears flowed down her cheeks. It seemed confusing to her because she didn't even know why she was crying. Her anger of earlier in the day had now subsided, but by no means did she think things were all right again or even marginally normal. She really didn't know what to think.

After getting Timmy a can of juice and giving Terry half of a Popsicle with a paper towel wrapped around the stick, Sueann went to the drawer in the kitchen where the telephone directory was kept and looked under "Psychologists /Counselors" in the yellow pages where she found a small boldface ad for "Newman Scott, PhD., MSW, Christian Counseling." She dialed the number and apparently a secretary answered, but Sueann was devastated to learn that Dr. Scott was fully booked up for new appointments until late next month.

"Please," Sueann asked the secretary. "I desperately need something sooner. I was referred to Dr. Scott by Professor Hargrave at the University. He recommended I call."

"Just a minute," the secretary said abruptly, placing Sueann on hold. As she waited, Sueann could hear a soft instrumental playing a variation of "*What a Friend We Have in Jesus*" on the hold function, which sounded vaguely funereal. She quickly wondered whether Dr. Scott was perhaps not the best choice of counselor under the circumstances, but just as quickly dismissed the thought. After all, Professor Hargrave had recommended him, and Dr. Scott had allegedly helped his daughter.

"If 8:30 in the morning is not too inconvenient, Dr. Scott can see you then," the secretary announced in a rather irritated voice after coming back on the line.

"That's fine – I can make it," Sueann answered without hesitation.

That night, when Sueann went to bed at nine Tom had still not come home, and Sueann did not hear him come in during the night. However, the next morning at seven Tom was already dressed and sitting at the breakfast nook table when Sueann came into the kitchen.

"Sueann," said Tom in a pleading voice getting up from the table.

"Not now, Tom," Sueann interrupted. "I'm not ready to talk, and anyway I have an appointment this morning with a counselor. In fact, it's a counselor Professor Hargrave recommended to us. Maybe you don't think you need a counselor, but quite frankly *I'm* going crazy because of you, and on behalf of *us* I need to talk with someone with professional insight into what is going on. I want you to watch the boys. I should be back by ten or so, and anyway you only have the one afternoon class today."

"Sure," Tom said without smiling. "Sue, can't I just say a couple of quick things before you leave?"

"No," replied Sueann curtly. "Not now."

Dr. Newman Scott leaned back into his black leather and chrome chair and pushed it on its coasters a bit away from his desk. He was a slender tall man in what appeared to be his mid-forties with thinning salt and pepper hair, the trace of a thin mustache on his upper lip, and a slight twitch in the corner of his right eye. He was dressed in black uncreased trousers with a dark blue web belt, gold socks, a short sleeve white patterned polyester shirt, and a black and gold sports tie imprinted with "Go Hawkeyes!" on it. Around the office were a framed jersey and several items on end tables and mounted on the walls obviously representing the University of Iowa basketball program, but none of the individuals depicted in the three or four matted photographs on the wall appeared to be Dr. Scott.

"Well, you certainly describe a fundamental breakdown in marital communication," Dr. Scott began after listening to Sueann's description of events over the last year and especially the last few days. "And without a doubt your husband Tom has been untruthful with you to at least some extent. However, I would not jump to the conclusion that Tom has been sexually unfaithful with this Glenda person."

"Gloria," Sueann corrected. "Her name is Gloria."

"Well," Dr. Scott continued, "the essence of Christian interaction – and especially for those in the more or less fundamentalist or evangelical churches which I take this Church in the Fields to be – is the idea of Christian love, and that love imagery is the idiom of a lot of church members' interpersonal communications. You can see that thematically in some of the passages of your husband's book that you just read me. This love theme is not a reference to erotic love, but rather to the agape concept of the spiritual commandment to love the essence of who a person is regardless of how ostensibly unlovable one might act."

"Yes, I know," replied Sueann. "But he's been untruthful about going to the church in the first place. It's natural to wonder what else he is hiding."

Dr. Scott smiled and shrugged his shoulders. "The basic handicap I am under is that Tom is not my client, and as I understand it, he refuses to see a counselor. Without an in-depth discussion with him and perhaps the administration of some standardized tests there is no way I could get enough background on Tom to make an educated Axis 1 diagnosis – if indeed he is even suffering from some kind of emotional or psychological condition that needs to be addressed."

"Look, Mrs. Schmidt," Dr. Scott continued, "It is very possible Tom is just going through what we would call 'a phase' if a much younger adult was involved. In fact, though, as adults get into their late thirties and early forties, they characteristically begin to increasingly think more about spiritual matters. Maybe the Episcopal Church is, or at least by Tom's way of reckoning has been, too superficial – or not intense enough, let's put it that way – to challenge him to grow spiritually. I certainly agree with Professor Hargrave that Tom's book is a poor example of *academic* research, but on the other hand it may be chock full of spiritual insights and may well be publishable in other contexts and on other aisles of the bookstore. I don't know. And as far as his apparent obsession with the 'uncreated light' theme, you should know that light, the sun, enlightenment, and things of this nature are all ancient idioms for God in the Christian iconography. 'God is light,' says the Apostle John in his first letter. There are probably other examples I don't know about. So, I wouldn't really ascribe too much of a problem area to his terminology about light and God. As for God talking to him, I would think that most Christians at some time or another believe that God has communicated to them in some way. I'm not the least bit hesitant in telling you that I firmly believe God guided me in graduate school more years ago than I would care to think about to become a Christian counselor."

"Did he tell you to write a book and then dictate to you what to write?" asked Sueann somewhat put off.

"No, he didn't do that," replied Dr. Scott.

"So, what you're saying is just to go home and forget about it," said Sueann.

"No, that *not* what I am saying," replied Dr. Scott. "In fact, I have some very specific things I would like to see you do. First, despite the fact that the truth of Tom's recent religious activities came out in a way suggesting deception on his part, I would like you to keep an open mind on what this is all about and more importantly Tom's motivations in possibly seeking a stronger religious experience than maybe your present church family is offering at this time. Secondly, I would like you to consider asking Tom to take you to one of these services he has been going to at the Church in the Fields. I am not suggesting that it was proper for Tom to go to the church without at least your knowledge or that you need to change church affiliations for any reason you yourself do not actively desire. However, I think it would do you a world of good to see for yourself and firsthand what this church is all about, and perhaps in the process you will get some insight into your husband's desire to go there. You may not like what you see, but I am fairly sure no one will jump out at you or make you uncomfortable. Christians are a pretty passive bunch generally. Thirdly, I would like for you to seek a physician who is experienced in treating anxiety and maybe the beginning stages of depression. Tom is not my client. You are, and I am concerned that the stress of the last few months especially has taken a toll on your emotional being. A well-respected colleague of mine who can size up these indications I am getting from a medical standpoint is Dr. Gerald Feingold. Dr. Feingold is one of four practicing psychiatrists in Madisonville. He doesn't have that many private patients due to his work at the Northwest Iowa Hospital, but if you allow me to, I will call him and get you an appointment."

"So, Tom takes dictation from God, won't eat meat, and goes to a fundamentalist church in a corn field, but you think I'm the one who needs a psychiatrist," Sueann replied flatly.

"No, Mrs. Schmidt, that is not what I am saying. *You* are my client. Your husband is not. I am worried about your husband only in as much as it may have an effect on you. But I am directly and professionally concerned about *your* emotional health based on our conversation this morning. Check it out medically – that's all I'm saying. Your children don't need a stressed-out mother at the same time you are struggling to make some sense out of your husband's behavior."

Sueann sat silent for a few seconds.

"All right?" asked Dr. Scott. "Does that sound reasonable?"

"I suppose so," answered Sueann with a deep breath.

"Then I'd like to see you back here after your appointment with Dr. Feingold in two weeks. I think this is going to work out. Who knows, you might actually find the Church in the Fields service meaningful to you in a way you did not expect. We'll talk about the experience hopefully next time. The initial consultation fee is $70.00. I'm sorry, but unless it's a health insurance program I am unfamiliar with, I don't believe insurance will pay for the visit. Angelle, my secretary will give you an appointment, and we'll call you as to Dr. Feingold's availability later on today."

Chapter Fourteen

By the time Sueann got home Tom was waiting with a message that Dr. Scott's office had called and confirmed an appointment for her with Dr. Feingold for Saturday a week, 10 o'clock a.m., at his Madisonville Office located in the Doctor's Annex next to St. Elizabeth Hospital on the Medical Loop.

"Are you O.K.?" Tom asked her as she laid Tom's book and her purse down, took the message Tom had scribbled, and posted it on the refrigerator under the rooster magnet. "Another doctor? I'm worried about you."

"That's a switch," replied Sueann. "Maybe it's time you worried about your family a little."

"Tom," Sueann continued, "why did you submit that ridiculous book to Dr. Hargrave and start so much trouble? Is that really what you have been working on for months?"

"I know you don't understand," replied Tom sympathetically. "No one understands. I didn't even understand until . . ." Tom fell silent and turned his head away to look out of the kitchen window.

"Until what?" asked Sueann. "What made you understand?"

Tom continued to look out of the window silently and lightly shook his head back and forth negatively.

"Tom," continued Sueann on a different tack. "Are the services at the Church in the Fields on Saturday like the article I read last year said?"

"Yes," said Tom flatly still staring out of the window.

"Then I would like for you to take me to the service day after tomorrow. It might help to clear the air between us. Sarah Jenkins can watch the boys for us."

Tom turned around with a broad smile on his face.

"Would you like that, Tom?" Sueann asked.

"Yes, we would like that very much," said Tom. "I was hoping I'd hear you say that one day. You won't regret it."

"Who's 'we' Tom?" Sueann asked. "You and Gloria?"

"No," said Tom flatly as he turned and began to walk into the den. "I told you Gloria is just a friend."

When Sueann emerged from the bedroom with Terry in tow on Saturday morning she found Tom already dressed drinking a glass of water with his blanket and pillow neatly folded and stacked at one corner of the divan.

"Do you still want to go to Shabbat service?" asked Tom.

"Sure," said Sueann as she lifted Terry up to the kitchen table. "What time is the service?"

"Ten," replied Tom.

"Well, that's over two hours from now," said Sueann. "That should give us enough time to feed the boys and get ready."

Sueann was silent on the drive to the church.

"Do you want me to tell you about the service?" Tom asked.

"No, Tom," Sueann replied. "I'd just like to see things for myself and draw my own conclusions."

"You'll like it," said Tom enthusiastically.

No sooner had the couple parked and got out of their car than people with enthusiastic smiles on their faces began to approach.

"You don't need to tell me who this is," one woman said extending her hand to Sueann. "Mrs. Schmidt we've been dying to meet you."

"So, he finally dragged you to our meeting!" Elder Dave Woods said.

Cecile Gates and his wife approached the Schmidts as they neared the two huge double barn doors of the church. Putting both arms around him, Cecile gave Tom an enthusiastic hug and kissed him on one cheek.

As Cecile's wife Gladys was hugging and kissing Tom on the cheek, Cecile extended his hand to Sueann and said, "welcome from the entire community, Sueann. My Brother Tom has told us all about you, and we've been praying for your situation for so long I feel as if we are already friends."

"What 'situation'?" Sueann asked with an embarrassed look on her face, but Cecile had already turned away and was in the process of extending hugs and kisses on the cheek to another nearby couple.

Just inside the large double doors, Sueann and Tom met Reverend and Mrs. Dykes in their usual station as greeters of the congregation.

"Well lookie here!" Reverend Dykes exclaimed enthusiastically. "Tom, you've finally had the decency to bring your better – and better looking – half to Shabbat Service." The reverend let out a huge and joyful laugh.

"Welcome," Mrs. Dykes said graciously to Sueann extending her hand. "In Jesus' name we welcome you, Mrs. Schmidt."

As Tom and Sueann made their way through several groups of people standing and talking in the broad center aisle between the rows of chairs, Sueann whispered to Tom, "where's Gloria? Show me Gloria."

"Ah, Gloria," said Tom looking around. "Gloria, Gloria – oh there's Gloria!"

"Hi Gloria!" Tom shouted, waiving to a woman seated in the middle of a long row of folding chairs on the left-hand side of the congregation. "Look who I brought!"

The smallish, middle-aged woman with mousy brown short hair smiled and waved back, and then cupping her hands to her mouth said something inaudible in return. Suddenly, the band began to play and the screen at the front of the congregational area lit up with the words of the first song.

> *Glory, glory, glory to the King of Kings!*
> *Lord, we lift up your name*
> *With hearts full of praise!*
> *Be exalted, oh Lord our God,*
> *Glory to the King of Kings.*

For the first thirty minutes the music ministry played, Sueann stood quietly and nearly expressionless beside Tom as he clapped in unison to the music and sang the words flashed upon the screen in front. During one last slower paced song, a group of ten women, ranging in age from little girls to senior citizens danced down the center aisle turning in circles and waving wreaths of some kind trimmed with colorful flowing ribbons. They were all dressed in ankle length lavender crepe skirts and were barefoot.

"Dance, women of God – dance for the pleasure of Jehovah Jireh, our ever-present Lord!" the music leader shouted into the microphone. Then teenagers carrying their fluttering flags streamed down each side aisle of the congregation and joined the dancers in a final assembly line in front as the congregation sang.

We are standing on holy ground
And I know that there are angels all around.
Let us p-r-a-i-s-e Jesus now!
We are standing in his presence, on holy ground.

As a hush fell over the congregation, and everyone resumed their seats on the folding chairs, Sueann heard a voice ring out towards the back of the meeting hall.

"Ja ka tra ka tra mee oobie ja!" a masculine voice rang out. "Jim ja kobe rah. Kobe rah, mo obbie!"

"Testify to the word of God, and interpret these holy tongues, Elder Tom Schmidt!" Reverend Dykes said into his microphone, rising from his chair in front and pointing to where Sueann and Tom sat.

To Sueann's horror, Tom rose from his seat next to her, turned to face the majority of the congregation and said in a loud voice, "Hear me, see me, Oh people of God. Use your hearts to hear and use your spiritual eyes to see."

"Praise God," one woman shouted. "Glory!" came other voices as Tom resumed his seat beside Sueann.

"You are an elder?" Sueann whispered inquisitively as she tugged on Tom's sports jacket sleeve. "What's an elder?"

Tom was silent and looked straight ahead.

During the sermon, Reverend Dykes walked up and down the center aisle of the congregation carrying his open Bible clutched tightly in one hand so as not to lose his grip when gesticulating with both arms to make a point.

"Beloved," the preacher began, "the entire bases of both the Judaic and Christian religious ethical foundations are based on *revelation*. I am told the same is true of the Muhammadan people who believe everything the so-called prophet Muhammad said was the revealed word of God and even the godless Buddhists who say that everything their little fat Buddha said on earth was true. You get the point. In these *revelation*-based religions the only basis for saying something is morally 'true' or 'ethical' or 'good' is that 'God has said it.' As people of the living God, we believe that the words of God in this book, both the Old and New Testaments, came both directly and indirectly from the mouth and tongue of the Almighty himself and are true. T-R-U-E true. This very simple proposition was hit home to me when I was praying over some passages in the Book of Joshua this last week that some ministers – some so-called ministers of the Gospel- have a hard time with. Now people of God, put down your Bibles and just listen to this. I can give you the references later." Opening his Bible, he read out loud.

> *But of the cities of these people, which the Lord thy God doth give thee for an inheritance,* **thou shalt save alive nothing that breatheth**; *but thou shalt utterly destroy them; namely the Hittites, and the Amorites, the Canaanites, and the Perizzites, the Hivites, and the Jebusites;* **as the Lord thy God hath commanded thee***.*

* * *

> *And so it was, that all that fell that day, both of men and women, were twelve thousand, even all the men of Ai. For Joshua drew not his hand back, wherewith he stretched out the spear, until he had utterly destroyed all the inhabitants of Ai. Only the cattle and the spoil of that city Israel took for a prey unto themselves,* **according unto the word of the Lord** *which he commanded Joshua.*

* * *

> *And the Lord discomforted them before Israel,* **and slew them** *with a great slaughter at Gibeon and chased them along the way that goeth up to Bethhoron, and smote them to Azekah, and unto Makkedah.*

* * *

So Joshua smote all the country of the hills, and of the south, and of the vale, and of the springs, and all their kings; he left none remaining, but utterly destroyed all that breathed, **as the Lord God of Israel commanded**.

"My people," Reverend Dykes continued closing his Bible and laying it down on an empty chair, "the one and only ethical and unvarying reality gauge we have as professed Christians is revelation from God through this Book. Jesus said '[w]hy callest thou me good? There is none good but one, that is, God; but if thou wilt enter into life, keep the commandments.' The *Ten Commandments* given to Moses weren't some kind of ethical argument or theory of ethics like hedonism or utilitarianism they teach at the university in town. They were instructions whose only moral authority was that the instructions, or commandments, came from Almighty God himself. I'd call that authoritative, wouldn't you?" The congregation laughed.

"God writes the rules!" Reverend Dykes proclaimed in a loud voice. "We might want to feel that the Ten Commandments are largely practical rules for living in community. We might want to think – and many lost souls have – that there is nothing at all wrong in making a good, satisfying little 'graven image' and then bowing down to it. The Romans had household gods and little shrines with graven images that the entire family gathered around for prayer. Aside from the explicit, clear, plain, and unerring word of God, that doesn't seem all *that* bad. For Christians and Jews, the only thing *bad* about graven images is that God told us not to do that. Do it, and you're going to die said the Lord."

"The Sixth Commandment is '[t]hou shall not kill,' which in Hebrew may be more along the lines of '[t]hou shall not with premeditation murder your brother *Hebrew*,' since capital punishment in the Bible was ordered by God and carried out for various offenses. However, what if God tells you to kill your son – your own little Bobby or Allen or Joey – just as the word," Reverend Dykes paused for a moment to emphasize the point, "came to Abraham? Of course, just as Abraham was about to do it – was about to kill his very own and beloved son – an angel came to him and called off the sacrifice. But what if God tells you to do it, and an angel doesn't come to the rescue? What about if God instructs you to utterly wipe out the Hittites, the Amorites, the Canaanites, the Perizzites, the Hivites, and – praise God – the Jebusites, just as the Lord God instructed Joshua – total genocide – kill them all and kill all of their children and old people? What about that? Does the word of God make so-called genocide moral or ethical or good? Not according to the New York Times. Not according to the homosexual-dominated Democratic Party in this country. But Beloved, Jesus answered this question "yes", because apart from God there is no good, and as Christians we believe there is nothing evil about God. Joshua in the Old Testament was a true believer. God spoke to him, and he acted upon it. That's what we are *supposed* to do as the people of God. Do we dare have an ethical system of beliefs that is contrary to what God tells us to do in the *Bible*?"

During the prayers following the sermon at the front of the congregation, Tom excused himself and walked up front with six other men who proceeded to face lines of people as they came forward. Sueann could see Tom placing his hand on various people's foreheads and saying things inaudible from her seat in the congregation. At Sueann's insistence, Tom and she skipped the coffee hour following the service. When their Volvo had left the parking lot and was headed south on the way back into town Tom was the first to speak.

"Well?" he asked inquisitively. "What'd you think?"

Sueann was silent.

"Sue?" insisted Tom. "What'd you think about the service?"

"Let me ask you something," said Sueann in reply. "You seem to be some kind of official in the church. An 'elder' whatever that is. How long has this been going on? How long have you been coming here?"

"A while," replied Tom.

"So, it has been Church in the Fields on Saturday and St. Albans Episcopal Church on Sunday mornings with the boys and me for 'a while'?" Sueann asked.

"Basically," admitted Tom.

"I think you and the people at the Church in the Fields are stark raving mad," Sueann said.

No one said a further word on the drive back into town.

Chapter Fifteen

For the next week Tom and Sueann were nearly non-communicative. When not at school, Tom continued his nightly vigil either in his home office or on the divan, and Sueann counted the hours until she could talk with Dr. Feingold the following Saturday. Because her appointment had been arranged by Dr. Scott's secretary for Saturday morning, that meant Tom would have to watch the boys in as much as Sarah Jenkins, the next door neighbor, was coming back from Waterloo that morning after celebrating her brother's seventy-fifth birthday and didn't think she would be arriving home until at least noon.

"Tom, are you O.K. watching the boys when I'm at my appointment this morning?" Sueann asked sipping her coffee.

"Sure. Of course," replied Tom.

"Tom, I want you to promise me that you will not be taking the boys to *that* church of yours. I have big problems with this church, and I do not want the boys taken there. Can you promise me that before I go?"

"Sure," said Tom.

"Sure what?" replied Sueann. "Sure you give me your word that you will not take the boys to that church, you won't go to the church yourself and leave them unattended, and you all three will be here safe and sound when I get back?"

"Oh, Sueann," said Tom with a disgusted tone of voice. "Don't be dramatic. Yes, we'll be here when you get back. Now, you'd better scoot. You need to give yourself thirty minutes to get to St. Elizabeth."

Nevertheless, as a nervous precaution Sueann verified that both of the boy's booster seats were in her car and not Tom's before she pulled out of the driveway.

"Come in, come in," Sueann heard a pleasant voice call through an open conference room door as she walked into Dr. Feingold's suite at the

Doctor's Annex. "My assistant Shelia is only available in emergencies on Saturdays, and I'm sort of 'batching it' right now."

"You must be Mrs. Schmidt," Dr. Feingold said as he emerged from the conference room. "Gerry Feingold, how do you do?"

Dr. Feingold was a pleasant looking, somewhat elderly, man dressed in what appeared to be the trousers and vest of an expensive brown-tone tweed suit, perhaps tailor made. His crisp long-sleeved white shirt with a monogrammed cuff was accented by a coordinated gold and rust colored tie protruding from the top of his neatly buttoned vest. He wore roundish glasses with gold frames, and every strand from his somewhat attenuated crop of light brown and gray hair was in place. Dr. Feingold's appearance and broad reassuring smile was such that Sueann was placed immediately at ease. "At last, someone a little bit normal," she thought to herself as Dr. Feingold showed her into the small conference room furnished with a large and small simple formica-topped table and blue plastic chairs ensemble.

"Well, 'here we are' as the saying goes," said Dr. Feingold sitting down. "I am at your disposal, and until I have to take my grandson somewhere at three, I have no intervening appointments. Why don't you begin at the end and tell me why it is you are here, and then I can ask some preliminary questions and we can fill in some details."

"Well," replied Sueann, "Dr. Scott thought I had anxiety and maybe depression, and . . ." For some inexplicable reason Sueann began to sob uncontrollably. Dr. Feingold reached behind him to the smaller table and produced a box of Kleenex that he gently pushed forward.

"Sometimes we cry a lot here," the doctor said sympathetically. "Don't worry about it."

"Let me ask you this," continued the doctor as Sueann dabbed her eyes. "How often have you been crying lately?"

"Some," sobbed Sueann. "I guess a lot."

"How long has it been since you had a good laugh or spent a pleasant afternoon in an activity?"

"I don't know," Sueann sniffed putting down the Kleenex in a wad on the table. "A while, I guess."

"How's your sex life?" asked the doctor.

"What sex life?" Sueann asked, smiling a bit for the first time.

"Sleep?" the doctor asked. Sueann shook her head negatively. "Not much," she said.

"Appetite?"

"Not much," Sueann repeated.

"Any unusual aches or pains?" the doctor asked.

"Back," said Sueann. "And neck. A lot of neck lately."

"You haven't thought of harming yourself, have you?"

Sueann shook her head 'no' and then chuckled out loud sniffing. "Maybe killing my husband, but not myself." The doctor smiled with her.

"Well, Mrs. Schmidt," said Dr. Feingold. "Right off the bat I'd say without going any further that you've earned yourself a prescription for a medication in the class of drugs we shrinks call serotonin reuptake inhibitors, or SSRIs. Serotonin is a natural secretion of the body – and specifically the brain – that takes the edge off a thousand little worries and headaches in life, and – when we chemically slow down the brain's re-absorption, or 'reuptake', of the serotonin it periodically secretes – many people report not feeling so low and emotionally out of sorts. They do not feel as depressed – hence the term 'anti-depressant.' But that's not really why you're here, is it, Mrs. Schmidt?"

Sueann shook her head.

"You know," said Dr. Feingold, "in my area of medicine prescriptions can sometimes help a little, but sadly they are almost never a total answer to a problem. Many times, underlying problems have to be addressed, and the root causes of an overall problem sorted out. Why don't you tell me in your own words why it is *you* think you are unhappy and out of sorts. You mentioned your husband. Was that a joke or is there something about you and your husband – or just you – or just your husband for that matter – that is troubling you?"

Sueann took a deep breath and exhaled. There was something about this well dressed kindly, older man that was putting her very much at ease. He reminded her very much of the way her grandfather looked and sounded when she was little.

"Yes, it's my husband," Sueann said.

"What about your husband?" the doctor inquired.

"Well, I don't know how to say it exactly," replied Sueann, "but he's turned into a kind of religious nut I guess."

"As I'm sure you know," said Dr. Feingold, "I'm kind of in the nut business. I love hearing about nuts. Tell me all about it."

Sueann laughed out loud at the doctor's joke. The last fragment of doubt she had about seeking professional help for the situation disappeared. She trusted telling this virtual stranger her story now, because on some emotional level he had touched her, and she was relaxed and trusting. In an instant Sueann's mind cleared, and beginning at the beginning, she told the doctor everything she could remember about her and Tom's religious experiences – both separately and together. The doctor interrupted very few times in the narration for clarification until she finished with the description of last Saturday's service at the Church in the Fields forty minutes after she began talking.

"You say Tom wasn't religious at all until a few years back," clarified the doctor, "and then he became increasingly intense about religious things?"

"Yes," replied Sueann. "Oh, I wish I'd never pressured him into going to church in the first place!"

"Well, I wouldn't worry too much about that, Mrs. Schmidt," Dr. Feingold said. "I'm getting the impression that if Tom had seen a political television show several years ago we might be talking about the Democrats and Republicans now instead of religion, or if he liked rock and roll music he might be talking about a new career in show business. These types of sensory intense topics can often be triggers for underlying problems, but they are seldom the problem itself. Let me ask you a few questions that might at first blush sound strange to you but might make a little more sense to someone on my side of the table. Has your husband exhibited any quirky tendencies lately in his daily habits – shifting from the routine. For example, in the clothing he wears, or perhaps in colors or areas of the house or your neighborhood he now avoids where he formerly didn't."

"Well, he refuses to eat any food that's colored yellow," said Sueann, "and our little washroom in the garage was painted yellow, but three weeks ago he came home from work one day with a gallon of white paint and repainted the room. Is that what you're talking about?"

"Maybe," said Dr. Feingold. "Why do you think he picked the color white to paint the room?"

"Oh, white is his thing," said Sueann. "White shirts. White towels in the bathroom to dry off with. White comforter and sheets on the bed. Even white food like plain mashed potatoes and cauliflower. Rice. It's about all he eats. He even threw a fit when I bought pale blue Kleenex. He uses a lot of Kleenex. He demanded that I take the blue Kleenex back and buy only white."

"Why does he use a lot of Kleenex?" asked the doctor. "Sinus problems?"

"No, no problems like that," said Sueann. "I really don't know why he uses so much Kleenex, but when I go into the office its trash can be overflowing with Kleenex that looks like he just pulled sheet after sheet out of the box and threw them away. They aren't even dirty."

"Interesting," said Dr. Feingold. "Tell me again about the book he wrote. It's a pity you didn't bring it with you."

"Well, he wrote in the book that what he calls the 'uncreated light' dictated the entire thing to him and he wrote it down."

"Maybe he was exercising a bit of poetic license," said the doctor. "Has he made any other references to receiving messages from people or sources that weren't visible?"

"No, not really," said Sueann, and then almost immediately she added, "well, wait a minute. Lately he has developed a really irritating habit when I try to talk to him of referring to 'us' – not me and him mind you but him and someone else, or saying 'he' thinks thus or so instead of Tom himself in first person. Am I explaining myself correctly?"

"You're doing just fine," said the doctor. "Any idea who else your husband is referring to when he says "we" and who is "he" if not himself?"

"No," replied Sueann. "When I have called him on it and asked what he meant, he's clammed up on me and wouldn't talk at all."

"How often does he clam up on you?" Dr. Feingold asked.

"Pssht," hissed Sueann. "The question is when will he talk. We haven't had a decent, sane conversation of ten minutes duration in at least six months. I take that back. Let's call it a year."

"And at this Church in the Corn Fields last Saturday they were talking about killing people?"

"Only if the Lord instructed you too, but the preacher or priest – whatever – claimed it was all laid out in the Bible."

"Is it possible that the so-called Lord is the other person with Tom's 'we' or even the 'he' Tom has referred to in your short talks lately?"

"It might be," said Sueann. "He has said that the 'uncreated light' and the Holy Spirit are the same thing."

"And what examples did the preacher in this church use in his sermon about killing people?" Dr. Feingold asked.

"Oh, Perizzites or parasites. Something like that," Sueann said. "Oh yeah, and the Abraham sacrifice business when the angel intervened."

"The Bible story when Abraham began to sacrifice his son Isaac?" asked the doctor.

"I don't know," said Sueann. "I only remember Abraham and the angel."

"That's not a very comforting story as far as I am concerned as a professional in this area of medicine, I must admit, Mrs. Schmidt," replied the doctor. "Does that example out of the Bible disturb you in any way?"

"I hadn't thought about it," Sueann said.

"Let me ask you a summary question," said the doctor. "If you had to pinpoint one main and predominant change in your husband's behavior in the last year – and you've mentioned several – what would that be? The Kleenex, the book, what?"

"Oh, I don't think it's any of those things," said Sueann. Those are all weird little things. I would say the biggest change that has come over him – besides lying to me like a dog – is just that he has dropped out."

"Dropped out?" asked the doctor.

"Yeah," replied Sueann. "Out of family life, of school functions with the boys, out of parties and barbeques in the neighborhood – hey, out of married life as far as I am concerned. He keeps to himself when he is home. He's a loner. He didn't use to be that way. He locks himself into his office, and I have no idea what he does when he is away from home. He's a drop-out of our life, anyway, that's for sure."

Dr. Feingold smiled at Sueann.

"How are you feeling now?" he asked.

"Oh, so-so," replied Sueann.

"Mrs. Schmidt," said the doctor, "I'm going to go get my script pad and give you a prescription for that anti-depressant we talked about, but I want to tell you right now that I am deeply concerned about what you have shared about your husband with me. I don't like what I heard you telling me, and it's troubling. Part of my duties involves the official evaluation of persons that come to my attention in need of significant psychiatric assistance, or if not assistance at least a proper evaluation to rule out significant problems. I'm not talking about you. I'm talking about your husband. I don't want you to get upset, but I would be remiss in my professional duties if I did not give you at least a head's up. You are not a physician, and you are, of course, not a psychiatrist. But I want you to know that if I had first hand observed and heard from your husband what you are telling me you observed and heard, it would be somewhat of an urgent situation for me to get your husband some professional assistance."

"He won't come," replied Sueann. "I asked him to go to a counselor, and he refused."

"I'm not talking about a counselor, Mrs. Schmidt," said the doctor. "I am talking about a proper psychiatric evaluation and possible treatment. Moreover, at some point in time – and one can never predict just exactly when that point is – proper psychiatric evaluation and treatment is no longer the option of the patient to refuse. It simply has to be imposed upon the patient for the patient's own good and safety, and for the good and safety of his family and even society."

"Doctor," said Sueann, "you're not saying Tom is some kind of threat to me and the children, are you?"

"No, Mrs. Schmidt," said the doctor. "I am not saying that – at least not yet. I've never met your husband. All I am saying now is that I am seeing a lot of red flags, and as a professional there are a lot of connections going through my mind based on forty-six years of past experience dealing with all kinds of illnesses. I don't think you are emotionally ill. I think you are clinically depressed, and there is apparently a glaring obvious episodic cause of your depression in the person of your husband. I'm not as optimistic about his situation. I'll be frank. I do not like that fundamentalist church he has been going to. I didn't like it when I read about it in the paper last year, and I especially don't like it after I heard about your experience. I will tell you outright it is no place for your husband to associate with. Pretermitting topics of religious theory and the politics of religion, he simply does not need to be around that type of stimulus in his current situation. Your husband does not need to be encouraged to see angels and hear prophetic voices in the wind. On the contrary. It appears that your husband is in sore need of re-establishing himself with a firm foot in reality."

"What can I do, Doctor?" Sueann asked concerned.

"For Tom, probably nothing right now. If this is symptomology of what I am thinking about now, it may very well – and probably will – increase until some kind of crisis in functionality occurs or until Tom decides to listen to you and get an evaluation. But on the other hand, I am going to tell you this plainly, and when you leave, I am going to make a note in your new file that I have indeed explained this to you. I want you to be exceedingly vigilant that your husband's behavior does not transform suddenly into something potentially unsafe for you, for the children, or for the public for that matter. I really don't think he needs to drive when he is upset, especially not if he is annoyed and certainly not with you and the children at any time if he seems to be acting strangely. He doesn't need to drink alcohol – not even in small amounts. He certainly doesn't need to be engaged in any potentially unsafe activities like hunting or archery or things of that nature. And moreover, if he becomes very irritable or angry, I advise that you stay away from him all together until he either collects himself or you can get some help."

"What's wrong with him, doctor?" Sueann demanded bluntly.

"I don't know for sure," said the doctor. "I've never laid my eyes on him. But at this point my duty is to advise you based on *your* narrative and appreciation of events over time. I am taking you at face value as I must. However, based on *your* narrative, I see evidence of active delusion. I see evidence of at least auditory hallucinations. I see inappropriate affect. I see marked social isolation and withdrawal. I see an impairment in vocational functioning at the university. I see a clear obsession-driven behavioral abnormality. In short, I see potential evidence of an undifferentiated type of schizophrenia with religious thematic overlay. I remind you none of this is confirmed and is based solely on our interview. However, if this were a medical school quiz that gave your narrative as a hypothetical case and a student wrote down what I just said – he would be entitled to an "A" on the quiz."

Sueann plucked another Kleenex from the box on the table and began to sniff into the hankie.

"Are you O.K. with what I just said?" asked Dr. Feingold. Sueann nodded her head.

"Then I want you to start taking your prescription as directed. Be patient; it might be more than a week until you begin to feel the effects of it. I want to see you back here in two weeks – let's say from today, same time – I'll give my assistant Shelia a note, and in the meantime if something – anything of disturbing note really – occurs at home that you feel is bizarrely unusual or that you cannot handle on your own, I want you to call my medical exchange number on this card. Day or night now. I've got calls at four in the morning for forty-six years. You won't be the first, and you won't make me angry. If you call every hour for three days, on the other hand, the exchange will block your calls, sort of on the 'little boy who cried wolf one too many times' principle. If I happen to actually be indisposed at the time, another doctor from my group will return the call."

On the way home, Sueann stopped at the Rexall Drugstore and waited for her prescription to be filled. She was in a state of extreme agitation, and she forced down one of the pills prescribed without water when she got into the car in the parking lot. She spoke to herself as she drove, repeating that everything was all right and the family would just have to work through whatever problems were presenting themselves.

However, when Sueann drove into her driveway Tom's Volvo was not there. When she rushed into the house, to her horror neither Tom nor the boys were there either. Panicking, Sueann began to think simultaneously of Dr. Feingold's cautionary statements and the idea that Tom had taken the boys to the Church in the Fields despite his promise not to. Pacing in the den, Sueann tried to re-assure herself intellectually and calm down. "No, she had been specific," she remembered. "Tom had promised." She reasoned that the three of them could be anywhere – probably getting ice cream cones at Baskin Robbins – although she would give Tom a piece of her mind when they got home for letting the boys ride in his car without their booster seats.

But, after twenty minutes of worry Sueann could not cope with the stress any longer. Grabbing her purse, she hurriedly got into her car and drove at the maximum legal speed north of town to the Church in the Fields. She began to cry in anticipation of the worst scenario her mind could conjure. Then, in a falsetto half-gasp, half-scream Sueann spotted Tom's Volvo in the parking lot as she approached the church from the highway and even before she turned into the parking lot. She pulled her car to an abrupt stop in the middle of the parking lot's gravel lane closest to the church's big double doors, threw open the car door, and got of the car without either removing the keys, grabbing her purse or closing the door behind her.

Entering the church hurriedly and in tears Sueann stopped briefly at the rear of the congregation.

"Oh God!" Sueann screamed as she saw to her horror that the two boys were actually standing at the front of the assembled congregation with Tom holding each of their hands. Reverend Dykes was standing in front of Timmy with the palm of his right hand pressed against the child's head in a manner that tilted it backwards as the preacher was saying into the microphone, "A most pleasing sacrifice of a contrite heart to God!"

With a hundred heads turned suddenly to look at her, Sueann broke into a run in her high heels up the center aisle to the front of the congregation. With tears flowing down her cheeks and a fearful look in her eyes Sueann pushed Reverend Dykes away from Timmy, slapped Tom's hand away from Timmy's, jerked Terry's hand from Tom's grasp, and quickly led both boys by their hands back up the center aisle at a quick trot.

Ushering the boys into the booster seats in the back seat of her car, Sueann instructed Timmy to latch his belt and she herself fastened Terry's. As she turned around and shut the back door of her car, though, the heel of her right shoe got caught in the deep gravel of the parking lot, and she twisted her ankle – actually breaking off the heel of that shoe. Sueann was ignominiously thrown off balance and down into the gravel, ripping the knee out of one of her stockings and scraping the palms of both hands. As she clutched the broken shoe heel and lifted herself to her feet, Tom suddenly appeared beside her and attempted to assist her by taking hold of one of her elbows.

"Sueann, what is the problem?" Tom asked solicitously.

Jerking her arm free of Tom's grasp, Sueann forcefully slapped Tom hard in the face and then stabbed at him once, twice, and then a third time in the neck and back with the end of the broken shoe heel.

"You goddamned fanatic!" Sueann screamed as she struck him. Tom himself burst into tears, and in a moment he had retreated back at a run through the big double doors of the church.

"What's the matter, Mommy?" Timmy asked as Sueann sobbed uncontrollably on the drive back to the house. A trickle of blood fell from Sueann's hand on the steering wheel onto the bottom of her beige blouse, and tears blurred her vision of the road. Upset and confused, Terry himself began to cry in the back seat.

"That's it," Sueann said out loud to herself as she turned onto her street. She determined in her own mind to go straight into the house and call Dr. Feingold's medical exchange number.

"Either this crazy bastard is going with me right now to Dr. Feingold or he is never coming around us again," Sueann said to herself again out loud to calm herself with the new plan.

"Mommy?" said Timmy from the back seat. "What's a crazy bastard?"

Chapter Sixteen

Tom sat silently on the divan as Sueann angrily spoke, gesticulating with her arms and pacing back and forth in front of the fireplace.

"I'm not crazy, Sueann," Tom finally said. "I may be enthusiastic in my life in the Spirit, but that doesn't make me crazy. Aren't I allowed to explore my own spiritual life on Earth to the full extent possible?"

"Not and mess with me or the kids, Tom," Sueann answered coldly. She was still obviously very angry. "You promised me!" she blurted out. "You promised me you wouldn't take the kids out there when I was gone!"

"I didn't kidnap my own kids," Tom said. "Being blessed by a well-meaning Christian pastor with their father standing right there isn't exactly treating children badly or failing to take care of them."

The doorbell rang. It was Sarah Jenkins from next door who stood silently in the foyer after Sueann let her in.

"I saw the car in the driveway," Tom heard Sarah say to Sueann.

"That's fine," Tom heard Sueann respond to Sarah. "I don't know how long we'll be gone. Thanks for doing this."

Sueann returned to the living room and picked up her purse and sweater from the coffee table.

"Are you ready?" she asked Tom.

"Sure – whatever," Tom replied. "Write your own ticket. This is more than a little embarrassing."

At the door Sueann stopped to give Sarah a hug.

"Thanks again," Sueann said. "There are hot dogs in the fridge and buns in the freezer. If they both eat their hot dogs, there are fudgesickles also in the freezer."

Tom walked past Sarah without acknowledging Sarah's look.

Sueann drove the couple in her car down Elm Street until Range Line Road and then west on to the Medical Loop. Neither she nor Tom spoke until they were in the parking garage of the St. Elizabeth Hospital Complex.

"Sueann, this is ridiculous," said Tom. "Let's go back."

"Tom," replied Sueann, "Last week I visited a clinical psychologist recommended by your own department head who was worried about you, and this morning I poured out my heart to a psychiatrist – a psychiatrist Tom! I have a prescription for an anti-depressant, and now I have a medical history that says 'consulted with a shrink because husband was driving her crazy!' If I can humble myself to get help for the sake of our marriage and the children so can you – that is unless you want to get out of the car right now and start walking, because I'm not going to put up with your craziness anymore."

It was after five in the afternoon before Sueann and Tom were situated in Dr. Feingold's waiting room in the Doctor's Annex and brought coffee by a younger woman who introduced herself as "Shelia White, Dr. Feingold's assistant." When Dr. Feingold emerged from the conference room door, he was wearing blue jeans, a sweatshirt and tennis shoes.

"Mrs. Schmidt," Dr. Feingold said, "I had hoped we wouldn't be seeing each other again this soon."

"How do you do, Tom," Dr. Feingold said extending his right hand with a smile and shaking Tom's. "Mrs. Schmidt, why don't you wait outside here for a few minutes and give Tom, Shelia and me a chance to talk."

In the little sparsely furnished conference room Tom took a seat on one of the chairs next to Dr. Feingold's assistant as Dr. Feingold closed the conference room door and seated himself across the table in front of a white legal pad and pen.

"Tom, do you know why your wife asked you to come to my office this afternoon?"

"Yes," said Tom quietly. "I think she thinks I am off my rocker with religion."

"Are you Tom?" Dr. Feingold asked. "Off your rocker, I mean?"

"No, I'm not off my rocker," answered Tom. "I am a sincere Christian – that's all."

"Sincere Christians don't necessarily have a secret religious life unbeknownst to their wives and friends," said Dr. Feingold. "Is that sincerity?"

"I have been telling Sueann *gradually*," said Tom. "She's very conservative. She's . . ."

"Concerned about you?" interrupted Dr. Feingold. "Do you realize that she is concerned about you, and do you know why?"

"She said the boys," answered Tom. "She said I was messing with her and the boys."

"Are you messing with her and the boys?" Dr. Feingold asked.

"No, I am *not* messing with my own children nor with Sueann!" Tom said angrily.

"You are aware, are you not, that the church you have been going to is a bit controversial here in Madisonville?" Dr. Feingold asked.

"I wasn't aware of that," Tom said.

"If I told you that Reverend Dykes was involved in a very unpleasant and potentially embarrassing lawsuit with his congregation in Minnesota before he came to Iowa and established his church outside of town, would that matter to you?" Dr. Feingold asked.

"That depends," answered Tom, "but I think I would like to hear about it directly from him and not from you."

"That's a fair answer," replied Dr. Feingold. "Besides, I would like for us to talk about you and not necessarily about other people except your immediate family. Do you remember the topic of the sermon Reverend Dykes preached the Sunday your wife visited the church – I'm not talking about today when she came to the church, but a week ago when you and she visited together?"

"No," answered Tom, "not right off hand."

"Wasn't it something about loving God to such an extent that you ought not hesitate in sacrificing your own son to God – killing him actually – if asked to by God?" the Doctor said.

"Oh yeah," Tom answered. "It was on Genesis Chapter 22. Abraham and Isaac."

"Sueann additionally remembers," continued Dr. Feingold, "that Reverend Dykes also said to everyone that the followers of Jesus had left their wives and children to follow him. Do you remember that?"

"Yes, I remember that," said Tom.

"Well?" Dr. Feingold asked.

"Well what?" answered Tom.

"Would you sacrifice your children if you became convinced God was telling you to do it, and do you think it was a good thing for the followers of Jesus to leave their wives and children to follow Jesus?" asked the doctor.

"I guess that depends," said Tom suddenly looking agitated with glances back and forth from Dr. Feingold to his assistant.

"Why would it have to depend?" asked the Doctor. "Depend on what?"

"Well, I'm not sure exactly," said Tom. 'I guess it would depend on . . ."

"On whether you thought God had *actually said it*?" interjected Dr. Feingold.

"For sure that," said Tom. "Maybe on other things as well."

"Sueann remembers Reverend Dykes touching one of your sons this morning when she was at the church and saying he was a sacrifice," Dr. Feingold said.

"He did not say Timmy was a sacrifice!" Tom retorted indignantly. "He was quoting scripture that a broken and contrite heart is a sacrifice that is pleasing to God."

"To be frank, Mr. Schmidt," the doctor continued, "he seems to be a very young boy to have a broken and contrite heart."

"He wasn't referring to Timmy," said Tom whose voice trailed off into silence.

"Tom," said Dr. Feingold, "Does God talk to you? I mean talk to you in a voice out loud."

Tom was completely silent.

"Tom?" Dr. Feingold asked again. "Does God talk to you?"

"I'm not going to answer that question," relied Tom.

"What's the big deal?" said Dr. Feingold. "Either he talks to you or he doesn't. Is there some problem in answering my question?"

"Even if he does, it's none of your business," said Tom sullenly.

"Tom," replied the Doctor, "It is very much my business – and I hope you understand that. It is your wife Sueann's business. It is the business of everyone who cares about you. I must also tell you that I am one of several Deputy Coroners for Hayes County. It is also part of my official business." There was a moment of silence.

"I'm going to ask you one more time, Tom," said Dr. Feingold. "And for purposes of this question I am going to go way out on a limb and assume that God does talk to you – at least sometimes in a voice you can hear and perhaps in some other ways. If God instructed you to sacrifice, and by that I mean kill, your own sons, or your wife, or even yourself – and if you were convinced that it was indeed the voice of God giving you those instructions – would you carry them out?"

"I don't know – I guess I would have to – Oh, I don't know," blurted out Tom. "It's a stupid question. God doesn't do those things."

"I thought you said he did," replied Dr. Feingold calmly. "I thought the Bible and Reverend Dykes said God did, and you agreed."

"Maybe sometimes. Maybe in history," Tom said.

"Would you like more coffee, or maybe a Coke?" Dr. Feingold abruptly asked Tom.

"Maybe a Diet Coke," Tom answered.

"Shelia," said Dr. Feingold. "Why don't you stay in here with Mr. Schmidt for a few minutes while I go and check on something. I'll bring us both back a Diet Coke."

Dr. Feingold closed the conference room behind him and sat in a waiting room chair next to Sueann.

"Mrs. Schmidt," he said, "I am going to be very frank and to the point with you. I believe you did the right thing in bringing your husband here. I believe he is suffering from a type of thought disorder we call schizophrenia or at least its affect. Now that's a big medical term and a scary one, but there are all different types of schizophrenia. Your husband's is apparently an undifferentiated type of schizophrenia with religious hallucinations and possibly delusions. I don't know yet. However, I am very much concerned that he could possibly pose a danger to himself, to you or to the children if he is taking his marching orders from a voice he calls God. I think he needs an extensive psychiatric work-up, and I think he needs to be away from the church he goes to *permanently*. Is there any chance of his voluntarily taking medicine and agreeing to stay away from the church without the necessity of a structured environment?"

"Well, he's lied before and slipped off to the church – and he doesn't think the slightest thing is wrong with him," Sueann said.

"Do I take it, then, that you think a structured environment will indeed be required for him to come to grips with his situation and cooperate with curative treatment if what I suspicion turns out to be correct?" asked Dr. Feingold.

"Yes," said Sueann, taking a Kleenex from her purse and dabbing both eyes.

"Will he voluntarily enter into a hospital for a limited period of time for evaluation and treatment?" continued the Doctor.

"You'll have to ask him," said Sueann, "but I don't think so."

"I'm sorry you have to go through this," said Dr. Feingold. "The emotional burden upon you is that under Iowa Law a psychiatrist is not customarily what the law refers to an 'interested person' for purposes of obtaining an order of Commitment for Involuntary Hospitalization. As Tom's wife, would you be willing to act as such an interested person on your husband's behalf – that is if he refuses treatment voluntarily – and sign an application that he be ordered into evaluation and treatment?"

"I don't know," said Sueann crying. "What do you advise?"

"I can't advise you, Mrs. Schmidt," replied Dr. Feingold. "That decision is yours. I can only tell you that if Tom was my father or my brother the answer to my own question would be 'yes'. I would sign the application."

"O.K. then," Sueann said sniffing as she put her Kleenex back into her purse.

"Well then here's what we should do," said Dr. Feingold. "I want us to be prepared if I discuss evaluation and treatment options with Tom and he strenuously refuses to the point of becoming upset. Then we would be in crisis, and perhaps a crisis of our own making. I am going to make three quick telephone calls and then rejoin your husband and my assistant. A person from across the street will come to the office, hopefully within the half hour and have you sign what is technically referred to as an application. If your husband agrees to a voluntary hospital admission, then no problem and the person will simply drive him to the hospital. If Tom does object, then he will still go with the person because the duty judge will have already pre-approved the involuntary hospitalization after I talk to him. Are you O.K. with that?"

Sueann nodded affirmatively with her lips pursed tightly together. Dr.

Feingold disappeared out into the hallway door, and after what seemed far more than ten minutes returned with two Diet Cokes, smiled at Sueann, and disappeared into the conference room, closing the door behind him. As Sueann sat and the minutes slowly passed she began to have second thoughts about the entire exercise. After all, she thought to herself, Tom and she had not really had a chance to talk about anything. Then she recalled her conversation with Professor Hargrave and the horrible look in that fanatical preacher's eyes this morning when he had his creepy hands on Timmy's shoulder and face. If there was a devil, she thought, she had seen it in that preacher's eyes this morning. "No", she decided, "something had to be done for the good of the entire family."

Sueann lost track of the time, and she hadn't even worn her watch that day in all of the frantic activity. Inside the conference room, which had been quiet, Sueann could suddenly hear a raised voice. It was Tom's voice, and he was yelling, "That will be a cold day in hell!" and "Not in a million years – my family needs me!" The door to the conference room opened about six inches, and then slammed closed again. Sueann had not been able to see anything or anyone inside. Just then the hall door to the waiting room opened and in walked two uniformed officers. One was a short gray haired, barrel chested, middle-aged man with a silver mustache, and his partner was a slender female officer with a big red lipstick smile and apparently long black hair which had been twisted and done up into a bun that protruded outside and behind her police cap. The female officer held a multi-page document of some kind folded into thirds, and she did all of the talking.

"Are you Mrs. Tom Schmidt?" the officer asked.

Sueann nodded.

"I am so sorry that you have to be a part of all of this," the female officer said. "It's always so difficult on the family."

"I'm Corporal Taylor," the officer said, "and this is my partner Officer Kenny Schilling. Are you O.K.?"

Sueann nodded her head up and down rapidly with her lower lip clenched between her teeth, but it was obvious that she was not O.K. Tears began to roll down her cheeks again. Corporal Taylor sat down beside her in a waiting room chair and put one arm around her shoulders.

"It will be all right," Corporal Taylor said. "You'll see. We want your husband to get better, don't we?"

Sueann nodded as she sniffed and took her wadded up Kleenex out of her purse again.

"I just need two quick signatures from you," Corporal Taylor said, unfolding the document and flipping over the first two pages as she withdrew a ball point pen from one of her uniform pockets and clicked it – here and here."

Sueann signed on the lines where the corporal pointed, and then the corporal rose to her feet, stuck the pen back into her pocket and rapped lightly on the conference room door with the back of her right hand and immediately opened it just wide enough to slip inside and close the door behind her.

Within seconds Sueann heard Tom shout, "No I certainly will not! You can't do this! I am an American! I have rights! Oh God, help me! Lord Jesus, help me!" Sueann rose to her feet in distress.

"Excuse me, lady," Officer Schilling said as he hurriedly brushed aside in front of Sueann and threw open the conference room door. There was a crash of clashing and colliding plastic chairs, and Sueann could see Tom leaning over the conference table with the side of his face pressed down onto the top by Corporal Taylor's right hand as she leaned over on top of him. Dr. Feingold and Shelia White leapt to their feet out of the way, and the force of Corporal Taylor and Tom's pushing against the table slid it over the tiled floor all the way to the wall where it collided with a crash.

"Don't hurt him!" screamed Sueann hysterically, but no one answered. In a scarce few seconds Officer Schilling emerged from the room pushing Tom ahead of him with Tom's hands fastened behind his back with some kind of black plastic band.

"Sueann, oh Sueann – how could you do this?" Tom pleaded, himself in tears, as Officer Schilling pushed him to, and then through, the waiting room door. Sueann burst into tears again and collapsed in a heap into one of the waiting room chairs. Corporal Taylor took a minute to adjust her disarrayed uniform and straighten her police cap. Then recomposing her wide smile, she sat down beside Sueann again and asked her, "did the doctor tell you where we are taking him?"

"No," said Sueann, "only to a structured environment."

"It's the Northwest Iowa State Hospital. It's north on Interstate 101 to the Williard Exit and then west on Iowa State 67. You'll see the sign for the hospital turn about ten miles west outside of Williard. It wouldn't be good to try and go there tonight. They wouldn't have visiting hours this late anyway."

"This paper," Corporal Taylor said to Sueann, "explains the law and the procedure for an involuntary civil commitment under Chapter 229 of the Iowa Code. There will have to be a hearing not less than 48 and usually not more than 72 hours from commitment. You will see where I have filled in the date for next Tuesday at 1:30 p.m. at the Civil District Court at the corner of Main and Post, Room 307. You will need to be there as the Applicant listed in the papers. An Assistant County Attorney, Nora Minden – long legs, green eyes, and red hair we would die for – handles these hearings and will be at one of the front desks in the courtroom. Just go up and introduce yourself."

"Will you be there?" Sueann asked plaintively.

"No, I won't be there," Corporal Taylor said as she smiled sympathetically. "You'll be O.K. – I promise. Are you all right?"

Sueann nodded her head and smiled bravely.

"I've got to run," Corporal Taylor said giving Sueann one last hug and rising. Nodding to Dr. Feingold and Shelia White, the corporal walked out of the still open door of the waiting room.

"Would you like to talk?" Dr. Feingold asked Sueann.

"No," replied Sueann. "I just want to get home to the boys."

"Mrs. Schmidt," said Dr. Feingold. "If you will wait a minute, I would like to give you a script for something additional to the Prozac. You've been through a lot today, and it will help take the edge off of the tension so that you can sleep."

Sueann nodded her head affirmatively.

"Shelia,' said Dr. Feingold, "get me the prescription pad off my desk, will you?"

Chapter Seventeen

"What's up?" a tall, cheery, slightly overweight orderly with short blond hair asked as he sauntered up to the night nurse's desk.

"Mr. Schmidt would like to make a call," the nurse said.

"And this somehow involves me?" the orderly asked mock dramatically by pointing to his chest with the index finger of his right hand.

The nurse rolled her eyes and indicated with her head in the direction of the back of Tom's chair.

"Oh, restraints," the orderly said out loud. "I guess you want the mobile phone."

"No kiddin' Sherlock," the nurse said sarcastically. "Pretty please with sugar on it help Mr. Schmidt with his telephone call?"

"Can't we just take these handcuffs off?" Tom asked plaintively. "They're cutting into my wrists, and some of my fingers are numb."

"I'm sorry, Mr. Schmidt," said the nurse. "In Madisonville those are handcuffs and can be taken off at the discretion of the officers who brought you in here, but here they are called restraints, and a transfer restraint status cannot be altered without an order by the on-call doctor. Dr. Jaharta has been contacted. He will be here shortly. He lives here on the campus."

The orderly appeared back with a large heavy-looking dirty white mobile phone. "O.K., Daddy O, what's the number?" he asked Tom.

"It's in my wallet,' Tom said shifting to his left haunch and raising up on the molded plastic gray chair.

The orderly withdrew his wallet and opened it up.

"In front of the bills section," said Tom. "It should be on a green slip of paper."

"Pastor Kevin at home?" the orderly asked.

"That's it," answered Tom.

"Okee Dokee," replied the orderly punching in the number. When it rang, he held the phone down to Tom's right ear.

"Jesus is good!" the voice on the other end of the line answered. "This is Kevin Dykes."

"Pastor Dykes!" Tom said, almost desperately. "This is Tom Schmidt. Pastor Dykes, I'm in trouble. I've been arrested and sent to the Northwest State Hospital in Williard. My wife insisted that I go to a psychiatrist who questioned me all about my religious beliefs and attending the Church in the Fields, and then they arranged for me to be taken by two cops out here. I need help." Tom began to cry audibly.

"Wait a minute now," said Reverend Dykes. "Just wait a minute, Tom. There is nothing that has happened or that is going to happen that the Holy Spirit can't handle. This is sure pure dee baloney. Don't worry one bit. The Church will get a lawyer for you, and we'll get to the bottom of this. I think you are entitled to a hearing by law, and we will make sure he is there to represent you whenever that is. Moreover, Connie and I are going to get on the horn as soon as we hang up and get everyone on the prayer line in intersession so that we can get you out of there. Tom, it's not like this hasn't happened to Christians before. Prison, asylums, crucifixion, and death. With God's help we can have the victory. Now, Tom, close your eyes and bow your head right where you are, and we're going to pray about this."

The nurse and the orderly stared at Tom as he began to mutter into the phone "She, ga ga ba sham – oh thank you Jesus, thank you Jesus! Yes, Lord, your servant is listening."

After a minute or two of silence, Tom said "amen. Thank you, Pastor Kevin, bye," and he straightened up pulling his head away from the phone. As the orderly disappeared with the mobile telephone, the nurse pulled a form from one of the stacked metal bins on her desk labeled "Nurses Notes" and began to write.

In about an hour, a small, thin, dark complexioned man in a cardigan sweater, white trousers, a blue cotton shirt, and a thin black tie walked briskly up the corridor and came to a halt at the night nurse's desk.

"Admission?" the little man said to the nurse at the night desk.

"Mr. Schmidt, here, Doctor," said the nurse as she reached for a small stack of perhaps four or five sheets of paper and handed them to the man.

"Mmmm," said the physician glancing through the stack. "Where is the MAS?"

"Last page, Doctor," replied the nurse. "The other side."

"Oh, I see it – thank you," replied the doctor.

"Ah, restraints," said the doctor looking up from the papers and arching his head around to the back of Tom. "There they are."

Kneeling down to the level of Tom sitting, the doctor said in a heavy East Indian accent, "Mr. Schmidt, as you know you are currently restrained. It is reported that you struck a police officer and attempted to strike your admitting physician . . . ."

"He's not my physician," said Tom.

"Well, regardless," replied the doctor, "the point is that you have apparently been quite upset this evening. Personally, I hate restraints. But I also hate getting hit. Do you realize that you are here for the time being, at least, involuntarily?"

"Well, of course," replied Tom.

"Do you also realize that this is a secure facility and that the doors are equipped both with alarms and a system of secured latches?"

"If you say so," replied Tom.

"Well then," said the doctor, "if I can arrange to take these restraints off you, will you give me your word of honor that you will not try and strike anyone or run down the hall or anything dramatic like that?"

"Sure, anything," said Tom. "Just get these things off my wrists." The doctor nodded to the night nurse who produced a small pair of cutters, rose from her seat, and walked around to Tom in order to cut the police handcuffs off.

"There," said the doctor as Tom rubbed his hands and wrists. "There is a meeting room just down the hall to our left. Will you please follow me there?"

Inside the bare meeting room was a small formica topped table and three orange plastic formed chairs. Taking the chair behind the table, the doctor motioned for Tom to sit down.

"I have some standard information to give you, and a few questions to ask, and then perhaps you can go and rest a bit – it seems from the admission notes here that you have had a pretty exciting day."

Tom was silent.

"Are you aware that this is the Northwest Iowa State Hospital we are currently situated in?" asked the doctor.

Tom nodded his head.

"Of course, you probably know the day of the week?" the doctor asked.

"Friday," Tom answered. "No, Saturday. It's Saturday."

The doctor continued, "the information before me indicates that a person legally designated to be in a sufficiently close relationship to you to make such a determination – namely your wife – has authorized your involuntary hospitalization here for a period not to exceed three working days in order that an emotional evaluation and mental assessment can be prepared, after which you are entitled by law to have a hearing at the District Court downtown in order to further determine your status. At that hearing you are entitled to be represented by an attorney of your choice and present any relevant evidence you want to bring to the court's attention. You will have reasonable access to a toll free telephone between the hours of nine o'clock a.m. and four o'clock p.m. over the next three working days – oh, I see where the hearing is set for Tuesday – over the next two working days to make any arrangements you wish. Are you with me so far?"

"Yes," said Tom quietly.

"In the meantime, and beginning right now, we will evaluate your emotional and mental status ourselves over the intervening time until the hearing. A few things about those evaluations we will be doing. First, it's a voluntary process, of course. There's nothing forced here. But at the same time if you do not cooperate with the procedure your failure to cooperate and more particularly *how* that failure to cooperate manifests itself will become part of the record and will be part of the evidence the court uses in determining your further status at the hearing. Are we on the same wave-length?"

Tom nodded his head.

"Now, let's get down to business," said the doctor. After about forty-five minutes of detailed questions as to Tom's medical, social and family history, his eating, drinking, and smoking habits, his hospitalizations and medical treatment history, and many questions as to his relationship history with family, friends, acquaintances and even strangers that manifested certain behaviors, the doctor shifted the questioning to the topic of religion.

"Do you have a religious affiliation?" asked the doctor.

"Children of Yahweh," answered Tom.

"I'm not familiar with that one," said the doctor. "Is it a traditional Protestant Christian denomination?"

"Not really," answered Tom. "We worship Jesus, but it's a lot of Old Testament teaching."

"Why don't I simply mark the 'other' box on my form here, and we'll leave it at that," the doctor answered.

Continuing, the doctor said, "you are entitled by law to know that your initial qualifying diagnosis which led to your involuntary confinement for evaluation and emergency treatment was schizophrenia and/or schizophrenic affect of an undifferentiated type accompanied by strong religious thematic overlays. Do you know what the term schizophrenia means?"

"No," said Tom. "Crazy, I guess. They all think I'm crazy."

"Schizophrenia does not precisely mean crazy, Mr. Schmidt," replied the doctor. "We don't refer to people as 'crazy' here. Who do you think considers you to be 'crazy'? I'm using your term, not mine."

"Apparently everybody," replied Tom.

"Does anybody or group of persons ever reassure you that you are not crazy?" asked the doctor. "Do you have support from anyone who might suggest that all these other people are wrong and that you are not crazy like everyone else seems to believe?" asked the doctor.

"Well, yeah – maybe Gloria Singleton and Pastor Kevin and a whole lot of people at my church, but also the most important one in the world – in the entire universe – has faith in me," responded Tom.

"Who's that?" asked the doctor.

Suddenly, Tom straightened up in his chair and turned his head to look at the plain blank wall.

"Mr. Schmidt?" asked the doctor. "Who is that most important one in the entire universe?" Tom was silent.

"Mr. Schmidt?" pressed the doctor. Tom turned his head back around to look at the doctor.

"I need to run just a cursory neurological evaluation on you if I could," said the doctor. "I promise it won't hurt or be uncomfortable. May I come on your side of the table?" Tom nodded 'yes'.

"Now," said the doctor sitting down in the seat nearest Tom and facing him, "keep your head straight but let your eyes focus on and follow my finger as I move it here. And here. And finally here. Good. Now may I just touch both of your eyelids for a moment? Any pain in your neck or head when I do this?" The doctor straightened up.

"Now, Mr. Schmidt," the doctor continued. "In my sweater pocket I have a small rubber-tipped hammer. It is used to test reflexes by gently tapping on two or three places on the body. I would like to take that hammer out of my pocket and use it to test your reflexes. I promise it won't hurt. May I do that now?" Tom nodded 'yes'.

"Mr. Schmidt," concluded the doctor as he sat next to Tom with his legs crossed, "I know that you probably very much would like to be elsewhere, and that is understandable by my way of thinking, but I would like you to know that while you are here and in the care of myself and the other staff members you are perfectly safe. Nothing untoward or unsafe or the least bit harmful is going to happen to you. Do you understand that?"

Tom stared silently at the doctor.

"I am almost finished with this preliminary examination, but I need to ask you if you have the least bit – however small – feeling that you might be better off by simply harming yourself?"

"No," said Tom.

"Well, put this way . . . ," the doctor continued.

"I'm not suicidal, if that what's you're driving at," said Tom interrupting.

"Good, then," said the doctor. "I think that concludes our evaluation. "Would you please be kind enough to simply remain seated for a moment while I turn in your paperwork, and someone will be on hand directly to help you?" Tom remained silent.

The doctor took the few steps outside the open door of the conference room to the night nurse's desk and handed her the packet of papers back.

"Well, back to my movie unless my wife has fallen asleep with it on hold," he said smiling. "We have a new guest. Chlorpromazine, 25 mg orally 3 times daily with 50 mg at bedtime beginning now and daily thereafter. That should be sufficient to relax him, but there's also an order in there for Librium 20 mg, oral two times a day prn. Ta ta." The doctor walked down the hall toward the exit as briskly as he entered.

Within ten minutes a short black curly haired nurse carrying a small white paper cup and a styrofoam cup of water entered the conference room, trailed by the smiling blond-haired orderly.

"Mr. Schmidt?" asked the nurse. Tom simply stared at her.

"I'm Julia, the nurse in charge on B-Bravo Wing tonight. We want to show you to your room and get you settled. In the meantime, Dr. Jaharta has ordered you some medicine to help relax you so that you can get some rest."

"Is it a narcotic?" asked Tom. "I don't want any narcotics."

"No, no, no," replied nurse Julia. "This is not a central nervous system depressant. The name of this medicine is chlorpromazine hydrochloride. It simply has a very tranquil effect, and the doctor thinks you'll really benefit from it during your stay here." Tom took the two pills with a small swallow of water.

"There," said the nurse throwing the two cups into the lined scrap can beside the desk. Now John and I will show you up to where I hang out and your room is. Bear with me, it's a bit of a hike. This hospital was built a long time ago, and it has high ceilings and long, long corridors."

Chapter Eighteen

The next morning Tom struggled to wake up as he lay in his single, and quite narrow, bed in Room 101 on the B-Bravo Wing of the Northwest Iowa State Hospital. Groggily, Tom turned over and forced his tired eyes open to survey the scene. His windowless room was large with what he guessed was a twelve-foot high ceiling stained by the discharge of two air conditioning registers, one of which made a soft whistling sound. The room was fitted with two beds, but the bed opposite him was empty and stripped down to the aqua green plastic mattress. Next to both beds were small side tables, and a dark green naugahyde upholstered chair separated them. The wide light-colored wood door to the room was open with fluorescent light from the hallway flooding some feet into the room like a diffuse beacon. Tom stirred in bed. He was wearing thin gray cotton elastic-banded pajamas, and a light cotton blanket covered him. Tom's mouth felt very dry, and it was hard to swallow. The saliva simply wasn't there.

Suddenly, panic shot through Tom's mind as he focused back onto the green chair.

"My cloths!" he said out loud with a thick tongue. "Someone took my cloths!"

Throwing off the cotton blanket, Tom struggled unsteadily to his feet – losing balance a bit and falling sideways into the chair in the process. Regaining his feet and balance, he staggered out into the light of the hallway and looked around blinking his eyes. He couldn't stop blinking his eyes. To his left the hallway ended abruptly after a storage room door into a seating area with a large southern exposure plate glass window. Opposite him was a series of windows along the west side of the hallway twenty feet down to its intersection with a broad corridor. To his right and across the corridor intersection was an imposing-looking nurse's station, faced in pale green tile with plate glass partitions extending from the desk level to the ceiling except for a centrally placed open reception space.

Tom turned and began to slide and stumble his way toward the nurse's station, flapping his arms in exasperation. His legs were heavy, and he felt as if he had to drag each rear leg forward as he walked. Behind the reception space he could see two women sitting, apparently engaged in an animated discussion. A smiling man in a blue scrub suit top stood behind them. As he approached the window, one of the women looked up suddenly and rose to her feet. She hurriedly walked around the station partition to her right and in a second was standing beside Tom with one arm bracing him.

"Mr. Schmidt!" the nurse said. "Cindy, call the new LPN to help me. Mr. Schmidt is really unsteady."

"Someone took my cloths," Tom mumbled through a tongue seemingly stuck in his teeth. "I need my cloths."

As a young blonde-haired woman came running up and added her arm to the bracing procedure, the first nurse gently grasped the underside of Tom's left wrist. "Don't be alarmed, Mr. Schmidt," the nurse said calmly. "Your clothes are in the closet in you room, and they usually put your valuables in the little drawer in the table."

"Cindy," the nurse said turning to the woman still seated behind the desk. "I know it's early to be this, but he's 110, slurring speech and staggering. Call the medical exchange number in his chart and tell them there are signs of dyskinesia. Lupie and I'll settle him down."

"Let's get you back to your room," the nurse added, gently guiding Tom around. Then suddenly Tom's focus fell on a figure coming out of a patient's room down the east hall to his left. To his horror he realized that the figure was Father Ben Grey, the Assistant Priest from St. Alban's in town.

"Oh no!" Tom shouted as the priest looked up, and Tom struggled in vain to break free of the two women's grips.

About twenty minutes later as Tom lay with his eyes closed on his bed and the LPN Lupie sat in the green chair next to him casually flipping through an old copy of *People Magazine*, there was a light knock on the frame of the open door to the room.

"Knock, knock!" Tom could hear Father Grey's cheerful voice say. Tom turned to face the wall.

"How are we feeling?" the priest asked as he walked over to the bed and the LPN stood up.

"Would you like a minute?" Tom could hear her say. "I'm on the one to one so I'll just be in the hall." The nurse took the magazine and walked out of the room, leaving the priest to occupy her seat in the green chair.

"Tom?" the priest said gently. "How are you feeling, Tom? I almost missed you. I usually get all of the Episcopalians on the Sunday Visitation List, but I see now where they have you marked down as 'other'."

"Did Sueann ask you to come here?" Tom mumbled from the crack between the bed and the wall.

"No," replied the priest. "I didn't know you were here. I didn't even know you were feeling bad. We take turns on Sundays visiting all of the Episcopalians here and at St. Elizabeth, and I just happened to see you in the hall. They told me at the desk they thought you might be having side effects from the Thorazine."

"Thorazine!" Tom said in an alarmed voice, rolling over in bed. "Nobody said they were giving me Thorazine. That's for crazy people!"

"No, no, Tom," said the priest reassuringly, touching Tom's arm and shoulder. "No one has said you are crazy. You are feeling ill, that's all – in a way similar to, but also distinct in its own way from someone who might be having heart or kidney problems. You are being treated for just one specific type of illness – that's all."

"Father, I need to get out of here," said Tom.

"That's not a big deal," said the priest. "The reason they've put you in a secure facility like this is because they thought your state of agitation was so great that you needed a lot of close medical attention you couldn't get as an out-patient. As soon as the medication kicks in, I'm sure you will feel a lot better and then you can start discussing going home. In the meantime, all you need to do is relax and take it easy. That will go a long way toward getting you home to Sueann and the boys."

"But I don't need Thorazine," complained Tom. "I'm not crazy."

"Of course not," replied the priest. "But let's look at it this way. If I needed to know a point of Christian history for a sermon, I would be wise in coming to you for help. You are the expert in that area. If I needed – or even someone who loved me *thought* I needed – medical attention for even a minor ailment I would be wise to consult an expert in that specific area of medicine. Life is not simple. In fact, sometimes it's very complicated. We all would do well to trust that the experts we are guided to by loving hands will help us in a productive way."

Just then, the nurse who had first helped Tom at the nursing station walked through the open door trailing behind her the LPN holding the magazine.

"O.K., Father," she said, "Time to wrap up the jawboning. I need Mr. Schmidt for two little injections."

The priest smiled and rose to his feet. "Take care, Tom," he said. "I'll be back to visit later."

After the injections Tom fell into a deep sleep, awakening only for a groggy time or two before the next morning. From deep within a dream Tom heard a voice, "Mr. Schmidt. Mr. Schmidt, can you hear me?" He opened his eyes to the same duct stained ceiling and subdued light beaconing in from the hallway.

"Mr. Schmidt," the same voice as the dream repeated. "Can you hear me?"

Tom turned his head to the left to see Dr. Feingold sitting in the chair beside his bed. He was immaculately dressed in neatly creased charcoal gray pleated trousers with a matching vest and coat, accented with a cream-colored shirt and dark red tie. For some reason Tom's eyes focused on the doctor's shoes – medium brown lizard skin slip-ons with thin dark gray socks. Tom nodded his head not making eye contact with the visitor, still focused on the doctor's shoes. He could see a slight scuff mark just to the inside of the right foot. Otherwise, the shoes looked new.

"What time is it?" Tom asked.

"It's Monday morning," the doctor answered. "You slept a lot. That's good."

"I feel better than . . ." Tom's voice broke off.

"I'm glad," said the doctor. "You had us worried about you. When you first came in you were administered a clinically sizable dose of a type of medicine called chlorpromazine, popularly known as Thorazine. It has a received a bad reputation over the last few years – some of it not deserved – but in your case apparently very much deserved because of your showing quite early signs of a rare side effect known as tardive dyskinesia. It's unusual for a patient to show those side effects of the drug that quickly and we need to think about other things like seizures, but because of the early onset and equally early withdrawal – we took you off the medication immediately – I don't think there will be any lasting problems if it was TD."

"You don't *think* there will be any lasting problems?" Tom asked incredulously pushing himself up to a sitting position with his legs braced on the floor over the side of the bed. His head throbbed, and his mouth felt drier than it ever had.

"Are you nauseous?" the doctor asked. Tom shook his head 'no.'

"Dry mouth?" the doctor persisted. Tom nodded his head affirmatively.

"Very," said Tom.

The doctor reached behind him to the little table and poured some water into a styrofoam cup. Handing the cup to Tom, he said, "those are the two most common side effects we see with Haldol – the substitute medicine we gave you. Oh, we have seen tardive dyskinesia too, though not as much with the Haldol."

"Doctor, I'm more worried about the side-effects of just being in this place. This is the Northwest Iowa State Hospital for mentally ill people? I am right about that, aren't I? My grandfather used to call this place the State Asylum."

"Oh, that's going way back," the doctor chuckled. "Even before my time."

"But regardless," said Tom swishing his last bit of water in his mouth before swallowing it, "that's where I am, and the reason I'm here is that you and my wife think I'm insane."

"I don't think anyone is insane," replied the doctor. "Sanity and insanity are legal terms of art that the courts and judges and lawyers deal with in determining whether a person is considered of sound mind enough to deal with his or her own legal affairs. Those are not medical terms."

"Come on, Doctor," Tom snapped. "Nuts, crazy, bonkers, out of it, around the bend, cuckoo, bananas – I don't care what you call it. The point is that I am now a prisoner in the Northwest Iowa State Hospital because you and a person I thought I knew have reached a determination – the two of you have reached a decision – that I am not reliable or predictable or stable enough mentally to fit into your world outside of these doors. Isn't that right?"

"You're here," replied the doctor, "because an initial determination was made that – absent a full evaluation and at least some treatment to calm your agitation – there *was* sufficient preliminary evidence to fear that without intervention you were a threat of injury to yourself or others. Tom, I gave you the choice in my office. We could have done the medication and evaluation on an outpatient basis."

"Who gave you the right to evaluate me?" Tom asked indignantly. "And who gave you the right to medicate me? Not even Sueann has that right. I may not be in control of much, but at least I have the right to be in control of myself."

"Until you demonstrate that you might exercise that right to harm yourself or others," replied the doctor.

"Good grief!" exclaimed Tom. "Are you and Sueann so anti-religious that you think just because I worship God in my own way and in my own understanding that I am a candidate to go out and harm someone in the name of religion?"

"Or of God – look Tom, it happens every day," said the doctor. "A few years ago, over nine hundred members of the Peoples Temple Cult that started in Indiana died in a mass murder-suicide in Guyana. Last year in Wisconsin . . ."

"Yes, last year in Wisconsin the farmer killed his wife and two kids and then killed himself because the devil told him to do it," said Tom sarcastically.

"Not quite the story," said the doctor, "but you get the point. Professionals in my position take religion very seriously these days."

"Or maybe not seriously enough," said Tom. "You don't personally believe in God at all, do you, Doctor?"

"What I believe is totally irrelevant to this discussion," replied the doctor. "Tom," he continued, "don't hold it against Sueann for caring enough about you to want you to get help."

"Pssht!" responded Tom. "Some help."

"You're making my point by acting this way," said the doctor. "Why don't you simply cooperate with the process, bear with me for an hour or two . . ."

"Because I'm not going to do it!" interrupted Tom. "As a matter of personal dignity, I don't have to do it. I don't want to cooperate with the *process*. I don't want to *bear with you*. I am here because perhaps you, but certainly Sueann, think I am a religious nut of some kind and one that needs to either conform to society's norms or be locked up. O.K., let's concede for purposes of argument I *am* a religious nut, or a political nut, or a something-or-other variety of nut – or just plain nutty and like to talk to the grass and the trees. I have a right to be *me* however that shakes out. I support my family. I'm a good father and a good husband. One of my marriage vows wasn't that I'd always act like Sueann wants me to act or that I wouldn't have beliefs that embarrass her. They didn't stamp on my birth certificate that I was only welcome in this State as long as I didn't go to church at some kooky barn meeting in the cornfields. My kids don't get to disinherit me because they think I'm the 'nutty professor'. I'm just *not going to cooperate*. I heard what that other doctor said, too. If I didn't cooperate, you'd tell it to the judge at the hearing tomorrow. Well, go ahead. Tell the judge I was uncooperative because I *am* uncooperative. It's a farce that I am in here, but it would be a far greater farce and affront to my dignity if I were to cooperate with the farcical *process* that put me in here."

"I'm sorry your feel that way," said the doctor rising.

"Yeah, yeah," said Tom lying back on the bed.

"Do you want me to leave the door open?" asked the doctor as he turned around at the hallway. Tom said nothing, and the doctor turned and walked down the hall towards the nurse's station.

That afternoon Tom placed a call to Reverend Dykes at the patient designated phone in the hallway next to the nurse's station.

"I just wanted to make sure you knew when the hearing was tomorrow," Tom said to the reverend.

"Third floor, Civil District Court, 1:30, Judge Giddeon," replied Reverend Dykes enthusiastically. I've got it all down here. And we're going to come out in force, Brother Tom. We're going to be there for you. Don't worry now."

Tom hung up without the reverend remembering to pray for his situation. Afterwards, in his room, Tom attempted to call upon the Uncreated Light. However, no voice or feeling of the Light came even after Tom washed his hands three times in between his prayers. He felt very much alone in his room, so much so that he propped his door open before he fell asleep so that he could hear the indistinct, but still comforting, murmuring at the nurse's station down the hall.

Chapter Nineteen

By the time Nick and Sammy from Hospital Security came to pick up Tom for the ride into town on Tuesday, he was already dressed in the same clothes he had worn into the hospital the Saturday before and was seated impatiently on the chair beside his bed.

"Ready to take a ride?" Nick, the older security guard, asked.

"Yes, Sir," said Tom. "Let's get this over with."

As the white van drove out from the back entrance of the B-Bravo Wing of the hospital along the flower lined driveway to the highway, Tom looked back and got his first really good look at the hospital in the daylight. The three storied red brick building was faced in the center by two large cylindrical brick towers with conical roofs placed perhaps a hundred feet apart. Between the towers were a series of third story gabled protrusions along the roofline, giving the entire building a rather gothic appearance. Extending far to the left of the easternmost tower was the A-Alpha wing of the hospital, counterbalanced by the western B-Bravo Wing to the right. Behind the main building and connected to it via two identical rear towers at the back were the huge D-Delta and E-Echo wings extending to the south. Tom had no idea why the wings were labeled so oddly or how they differed – if indeed they did – in terms of patient populations. He didn't care. He just wanted to get out of this hellish place, and he had a good feeling he would be out after the hearing in court.

Just before the hospital road joined the highway Tom saw a sign indicating that the "Hospital Cemetery" was down a little lane to the right. A cold shudder went through Tom's body thinking that people would actually die in this horrible institution and have to be buried on the grounds.

"Ya know," said Nick half looking back over his shoulder as he drove toward the Interstate on Highway 67 just outside of the little town of Williard.

"What?" answered Tom.

"Ya know that it's gonna be O.K. – I mean, whatever the Judge says, it's gonna be all right."

"I don't guess I know what you mean," said Tom.

"Well, it's just gonna be O.K.," answered Nick. "I've been doing this for thirty years, and I've seen all kinds of things. It's just gonna be O.K. – that's all I'm saying. Things always seem to work out even when they don't seem to at first."

"Praise God," Tom answered still not grasping what point the man was driving at.

As the hospital van turned right off Post Street on to Main in downtown Madisonville, Tom could see a crowd of perhaps three dozen people standing on the steps of the court house – some waving signs with the writing pointed away from the street – facing a man at the top of the stairs with a bull horn.

It was Reverend Dykes, and beside him was another man wearing a wide brimmed white western hat, cowboy boots, and a lime green double knit suit with a white shirt and string tie. Across Main Street the church bus was parked in the municipal parking lot, and as the hospital van passed, Tom could see a big banner had been draped along the side of the bus proclaiming "Religious Freedom For The People of God." Tears of joy moistened Tom's eyes into a blur. They hadn't forgotten. The Reverend had been true to his word. Tom thought that this was his family. His true family. Just like the story about Jesus in the Bible when his kin had come to take him away from a meeting and he had said, "no – these are my mothers and sisters and brothers – the people of my group". They were truer than true.

"Dog and pony show," Sammy said to Nick in the front of the van, snickering. Tom urgently put his ear to the window glass in order to try and hear what Reverend Dykes was saying into the bullhorn, but he couldn't make out the words. The hospital van rounded the corner and pulled into the rear area of the courthouse off Adams Street, parking under the "Authorized and Police Vehicles Only" sign. Sammy and Nick led Tom to a rear elevator and up to a third-floor hallway where Tom was shown into a small garishly lighted room with a gray steel door and no windows.

Besides four orange plastic molded chairs, the room only contained one other item – a sign warning "Prisoners Found Possessing Contraband or Causing Disturbances Will Be Returned to Lock-Up." Tom looked at his watch. It was 12:45 p.m. At 1:15, a tall, thin Black man was placed into the room with Tom. He was dressed in an orange jumpsuit and wore dirty gray plastic flip flops without socks. His hands and legs were chained between metal cuffs on his wrists and ankles.

"Whats you got?" the man asked Tom.

"What did you say?" Tom asked. "I didn't understand you."

"I say, whats you got?" the man repeated in a demanding tone of voice. Tom could not fathom what the man was saying, and so he sat silent.

"Shhhhh!" the man said laughing. He lifted his cuffed wrists and rattled his chains at Tom as he remained slumped down into his chair.

"Boo!" the Black man said, laughing. At 1:30 two sheriff's deputies came and took the chained man out of the cell leaving Tom alone again.

At 1:45, Tom knocked on the inside of the door several times until it opened. A uniformed officer stood holding the door open halfway.

"What's your problem?" the officer demanded unsympathetically.

"I was supposed to have a hearing with Judge Giddeon at 1:30 this afternoon," Tom said. "I've been in here for an hour. I don't want . . ."

"The judge will call you when he's ready for you. Can you understand that?" the officer said authoritatively. "Are you here for the sanity hearing?" he continued.

"Sanity hearing?" Tom asked, taken aback. "Yeah, I guess that's what I'm here for."

"Then just relax," said the officer. The judge handles all his other cases first, and then he takes up the sanity hearings in a closed courtroom. O.K.?"

"O.K." Tom said meekly as the officer closed the metal door with a thick sounding 'click'.

At ten until three the metal door abruptly opened, and Tom rose to his feet. Nick and Sammy were standing outside in the hallway.

"We're on deck," said Sammy happily. "Let's go."

Tom was led into Judge Norman Giddeon's courtroom through a side door adjacent to the Judge's bench at the front of the room. As he entered with Nick and Sammy, Tom could see Reverend Dykes and the man in the lime green suit standing behind a large table to his left. Directly in front of him was a tall, slender red-haired woman in a beige dress suit standing at a second large table. Beside her sat Dr. Feingold, and beside Dr. Feingold sat Sueann who looked down when Tom tried to catch her fleeting glance with his eyes. Behind the two desks was a railing with a short gate that extended across the courtroom and separated the judge and participants of the hearing from a small gallery with benches not unlike the pews at St. Albans Church.

The gallery was filled to capacity with the supporters from the Church in the Fields Reverend Dykes had brought with him. Along the wood paneled walls were framed black and white photographs and two oil portraits of stern looking men, for the most part wearing old fashioned suits with shirt collars turned up or bent in wings like a waiter's tuxedo. Up front, on each side of the Judge's bench was a large framed document in script. On one side the large inscription at the top read "The Ten Commandments" and on the other side the title was "The Declaration of Independence". The Judge was speaking, and Nick touched Tom's arm briefly as an indication to stop for a moment near the inside of the door so as not to interrupt.

"I see a show about once a month at the insistence of my wife," said the Judge, "and that's about all the shows I can stomach at my age – you're not going to turn my courtroom into some kind of show, now are you, Mr. Lamonte?"

"No sir," said the man in the lime green suit. His hat was off and out of sight. "That is not our intention, your honor, and that will not happen."

"You're darn tootin' that's not going to happen," answered Judge Giddeon. Then, looking out to the gallery, the Judge said, "ladies and gentlemen, normally the courts of this State and all others that I know of are open for the public to attend and witness the proceedings. Open courts are one of the hallmarks of a free society. There are exceptions however, and this proceeding is one of them. Chapter 229 of the Iowa Code provides that an Involuntary Civil Commitment Hearing shall be conducted in chambers or in a designated private place with attendance restricted to interested persons and witnesses unless, for good cause shown, the court is satisfied that admission of the public would be in the best interest of the defendant.

In this case the attorney for this hearing's person of interest, Mr. Clifton Lamonte, has waived his client's right to privacy and asked for permission for you well-wishers to remain in the courtroom during the hearing. I will permit that as long as the bunch of you understand it is a privilege for you to remain in the courtroom during this hearing, not a right. We're here on a serious matter. This is not a circus and it's not a Sunday School. If I hear one peep out of one person in the gallery the whole bunch of you will have to wait out in the hall until the hearing's over. Do we have a deal?" Several heads in the gallery nodded affirmatively.

"And now, Reverend," continued the Judge. "Spiritual adviser or not, you're going to have to sit back there in the gallery with your flock. Lawyers, participants and expert witnesses only at counsel table."

"But Your Honor," began Reverend Dykes.

"Reverend," interrupted the Judge. "I don't want to be rude to you in front of your people, but if you don't get on back there to the gallery right now and let me get on with this hearing, this man with a badge standing right here to my left is going to take you away. Do you catch my drift?"

Reverend Dykes nodded and went to the back of the courtroom.

The Judge nodded to Sammy and Nick, and Tom was delivered over to the table and told to sit next to Mr. Lamonte.

"I take it you are Mr. Thomas Schmidt?" the judge asked Tom.

"Yes, Sir," answered Tom.

"All right, Mr. Bailiff," said the Judge. "Bring the Court to order and call the case."

The uniformed officer standing near the witness box to the front of the court lifted up a clipboard and announced in a loud voice "all rise – Oh yea, Oh yea, Oh yea, the Civil District Court for the County of Hayes, State of Iowa, is now in session, the Honorable Norman Giddeon presiding. Peace, quiet and attention to the proceedings are hereby commanded. No gum chewing, eating, drinking or newspaper reading in the courtroom is permitted. God save the United States of America, the State of Iowa, and this Honorable Court. Please be seated. Case number 89-0056, 'In the Matter of Thomas Alvin Schmidt.' "

"Counsel make your appearances for the record," the Judge said in a business-like tone of voice.

"Nora Minden, Hayes County Attorney's Office for the applicant Sueann Schmidt," said the woman standing next to Sueann. "With me is Deputy Coroner Dr. Gerald Feingold."

"The court is well familiar with Dr. Feingold," the Judge interrupted. "Missed your three handicap at the Charity Scramble last Saturday, Gerry."

"Duty and all that, Your Honor," replied Dr. Feingold, smiling.

"Mr. Lamonte?" the Judge said turning to the other table.

"Clifton Lamonte, Your Honor, for the defendant Thomas Schmidt."

"O.K. counsel," said Judge Giddeon. "This is a Chapter 229 Hearing mandated by the Iowa Involuntary Hospitalization Statute of 1975 and is being held not less than 48 and not more than 72 hours after the court issued an *ex parte* Order of Commitment of Involuntary Hospitalization on a good cause declaration supported by a presumptive Interested Person and by at least one health care professional with a recognized standing in the mental health care field in the community of the commitment. I understand the Applicant is the defendant's wife, Ms. Minden?"

"Yes, Your Honor," the attorney answered.

"Accordingly, the Court finds the Interested Person has standing to proceed with the hearing. Ms. Minden, in reviewing the record I did not find a Notice to the Patient Advocate or a Certificate of Waiver. Has the Patient Advocate been notified of these proceedings?"

"Yes, Your Honor," said Ms. Minden standing up. "I have both the Notice and the Waiver signed by Mr. Clarksdale with me right here."

"Hand them to the Bailiff, then," said the Judge, "and the court will receive them into evidence at this time."

Continuing, the Judge said, "counsel, pursuant to the Iowa Involuntary Hospitalization Statute as expounded upon by the Iowa Supreme Court in *O'Connor versus Donaldson*, the court appreciates its task in this hearing as follows, and I am quoting now from the Judicial Bench Book approved by the State Bar Association:

> *The court's role is to determine whether or not by a measure of clear and convincing evidence the defendant is presently suffering*

*from a serious mental impairment which is defined as such an impairment that predisposes the defendant to the making of otherwise responsible decisions without sufficient judgment that characterizes an unimpaired individual **and** which impairment predisposes the defendant to (1) physical or emotional injury to such person's self or others **or** (2) fail to care for such person's own needs.*

"Call your first witness, Ms. Minden," the Judge said.

"Your Honor," said Mr. Lamonte standing. "May we have a brief opening statement?"

"I've read the pleadings, Mr. Lamonte," replied the Judge. "Is this opening statement calculated to be helpful to me or to appeal to the gallery?"

"You, of course, Your Honor," replied the lawyer.

"Make it brief," said the Judge.

"Your Honor," began Mr. Lamonte, "We would like to persuade the court this afternoon that this is not the usual case of this type your Honor sees."

"They're all different, Mr. Lamonte," the Judge said, "but proceed. How is this case different according to you?"

"It's different, Your Honor," said Mr. Lamonte, "because this case deals with the thin line separating the exercising of non-conforming religious practices guaranteed by the First Amendment to the United States Constitution and behavior that State Law might otherwise classify as 'impaired' under the statute. . ."

"I'm going to object to that," said Ms. Minden, rising. "Your Honor, if Mr. Lamonte is raising the lack of constitutionality of the statute for the first time during the hearing itself, I would move to strike that defense on grounds of lack of notice as required by the Code of Practice."

"Hold on, hold on, Ms. Minden," said the Judge. "Mr. Bailiff, hand me the record if you wouldn't mind." After three or four minutes of flipping through the pages of the manila folder handed to him by the Bailiff, the Judge continued. "I see no responsive pleadings at all in the file, but of course no responsive pleadings are required in a Chapter 229 Hearing because it is a summary proceeding. I suppose you are arguing, Ms. Minden, that despite the fact that responsive pleadings are not required in this matter, notice of the unconstitutionality of a State statute is required under the Code of Practice, so any defense along these lines appearing without written notice should be struck."

"Yes, Your Honor," said the lawyer.

"And I suppose you are arguing, Mr. Lamonte," continued the Judge, "that if an answer is not required in a special proceeding then the raising of a special defense such as the unconstitutionality of a State statue is not required prior to trial?"

"Yes, Your Honor," said Mr. Lamonte.

"A pox on you both," replied the Judge, "for making an old man use his brain after a big lunch. Mr. Bailiff, where is Caroline?"

The Bailiff moved over in front of the Judge and whispered something. The Judge scribbled a note on a legal pad in front of him, ripped off the page, and handed it to the Bailiff. "Tell her within the hour," the Judge said to the Bailiff, and the officer disappeared out of the same door Tom had entered a few minutes before.

"Subject to the objection, continue, Mr. Lamonte," the Judge commanded.

"The point is, Your Honor," continued Mr. Lamonte, "that we live in an extremely diverse society with equally diverse religious beliefs. If, for example, a prospective State Hospital patient in – let's say – a South Seas Polynesian society were to go around claiming he had eaten the body and drank the blood of the one true God, then he might well be bound and placed into an island mental institution, and rightfully so, because this same hypothetical Polynesian society had never been visited by a Christian missionary."

"However, had the same utterance been made at the Sven's Cafeteria here in Madisonville by an individual having just come from St. Aloysius Roman Catholic Church at Sunday Mass then the comment would be orthodox and non-objectionable. So here, a new church opens its doors north of Madisonville in the middle of the corn fields teaching that *both* the Old and New Testaments of the Bible are authoritative and binding on the faithful, and true and faithful Episcopalian Associate Professor Schmidt – who happens to be a historian and a Christian historian at that

– happens to embrace these beliefs and the next thing he knows he is on a ward at the State Hospital and declared mentally impaired. Imagine that!"

"Oh, I love it," said the Judge, "and imagine I thought my day was to be confined to six divorces, two pre-trials and a sentencing. Well, Ms. Minden, what do you have to say to that?"

"Oh, Your Honor," said the young woman rising from counsel table, "all of these arguments sound good from counsel. But we are here to examine the mental capacity of a specific person – Mr. Schmidt – not his counsel, however clever he might at first appear. We are not here to argue religion or philosophy. We are here to evaluate the mental capacity of a specific man in a specific context. Mr. Lamonte seems to be anticipating that your honor will find Mr. Schmidt is mentally impaired to the point of failing to make responsible decisions . . ."

"I am not making such a concession!" Mr. Lamonte said indignantly rising to his feet.

"Mr. Lamonte," said the Judge, "your opponent was courteous while you spoke. Do her the reciprocal courtesy and sit down." Mr. Lamonte sat down.

"As I was saying, Judge," Ms. Minden continued, "the key as the State sees it to this case is whether the evidence will show that Mr. Schmidt poses a danger of "physical or emotional injury to such person's self or others" as required under the Statute. Now, the State contends that it makes no difference – and I'll say statutorily or constitutionally – whether your thing is being a Republican or a Democrat or a Baptist or a Catholic or a Free Mason or a Woodsman of the World, the point *is* that if you quote – *pose a physical or emotional injury to yourself or another* – end quote then you need, and the State needs, the protection afforded by Chapter 229. That's the State's answer to the 'we're Americans and we can believe what we want to' argument."

"Well," said the Judge, "with that, call your first witness, Ms. Minden."

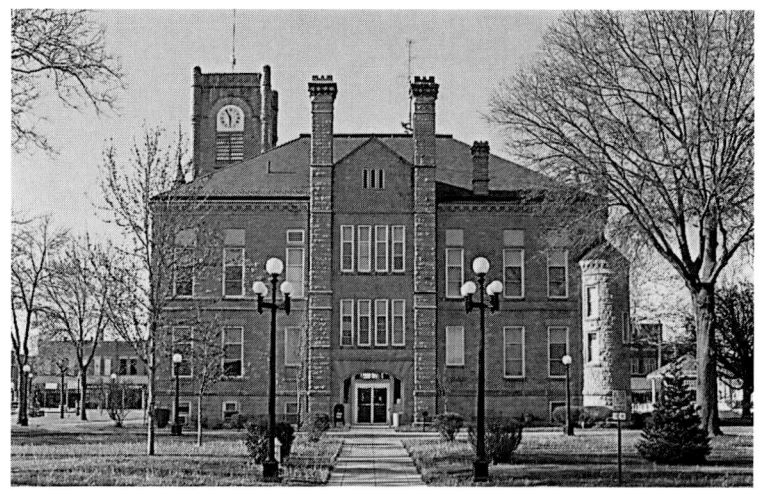

Chapter Twenty

The attorney for the State, still on her feet, said, "The State calls Dr. Gerald Feingold." The doctor made his way to the witness stand and raised his right hand in anticipation of the administration of the oath.

"State your full name for the record, please," said Ms. Minden.

"Gerald Feingold," was the response.

"Your Honor," said Ms. Minden, "the State tenders Dr. Feingold as a well-respected expert in the practice of medicine with a specialty in the area of psychiatry."

"Just one question?" said Mr. Lamonte rising.

"Save your breath," said the Judge. "Dr. Feingold has qualified as an expert many times in this court."

"One question?" asked the lawyer.

"If you must," replied the Judge.

"Doctor are you a Christian?" asked Mr. Lamonte.

"I object!" said Ms. Minden, rising.

"I'll permit it," said the Judge.

"No," answered Dr. Feingold.

"The court finds Dr. Feingold well qualified as an expert witness in the areas tendered," said the Judge. "Continue, Ms. Minden."

"Dr. Feingold," asked Ms. Minden, "are you now and have you been since the time of diagnosis the attending psychiatrist of Mr. Schmidt?"

"Yes," answered the doctor.

"And have you reached a professional initial diagnosis of any psychiatric illnesses, if any, which Mr. Schmidt is laboring under?"

"I have," replied the doctor.

"Doctor," asked Ms. Minden, "would you please tell the court what your diagnosis of Mr. Schmidt is?"

"Undifferentiated schizophrenia with a religious thematic overlay," replied the doctor.

"Has your initial diagnosis been confirmed, Doctor?" asked Ms. Minden.

"No," replied the doctor.

"And why not?" asked the lawyer.

"Because," answered the doctor, "of lack of cooperation and compliance on the part of the patient."

"The patient being Mr. Schmidt?" asked the lawyer.

"Yes," replied the doctor.

"Doctor," asked the lawyer, "is lack of cooperation and lack of compliance in medical requests an element in a diagnosis of schizophrenia?"

"Often," replied the doctor.

"Doctor," replied Ms. Minden, "in your professional opinion, is Mr. Schmidt seriously mentally impaired such that he lacks sufficient judgment to make responsible decisions for himself?"

"Yes," replied the doctor. "Based on current information."

"Does Mr. Schmidt's condition," continued Ms. Minden, "lead you to conclude that his presumed illness either predisposes him to injury to himself or others or incapacitates him from caring for himself?"

"Yes," replied the doctor. "Again, based on current information."

"Your witness," said Ms. Minden.

"Doctor Feingold," said Mr. Lamonte rising, "if I were to say to you that I believed the Lord God made the sun stand still at the Battle of Gibeon for twenty-four hours while the People of Israel made war upon the five Amorite Kings of Jerusalem, Hebron, Jarmuth, Lachish and Eglon, and that I believed the Lord God assisted the People of Israel in their enterprise by casting great stones upon the armies of the five kings from heaven, would you declare me stark raving mad?"

"No," replied the doctor.

"And why not?" asked the lawyer. "That sounds pretty incredible to me."

"Because that is a popular religious myth in the Judeo-Christian culture," said the doctor. "I believe you are retelling the story found in the Biblical Book of Joshua."

"As a matter of fact, I am, Doctor," replied the lawyer. "But I'm interested in knowing what, in your professional opinion, separates the people who believe in that myth as you call it from those living peacefully here in Madisonville and those inmates at the Northwest Iowa State Hospital."

"The subjective belief, Mr. Lamonte," said the doctor, "in what is a religious myth and what constitutes reality."

"Oh, come on, Doctor," Mr. Lamonte forcefully replied. "I can count on all my fingers on both hands the churches and denominations in this town that believe in the complete, inspired, and literal truth of the Bible. Count with me," he said holding up both hands and folding back each finger one-by-one as he spoke, "the Catholics, the Baptists, the Presbyterians, the Seventh Day Adventists, the Nazarenes, the Full Gospels, the Assemblies of God, the Lutherans – that's the Missouri and the American Synods – the Free Will Methodists, and the United Pentecostals. Oops! I've run out of fingers, Doctor, and I haven't even got to the Children of Yahweh and the Church in the Fields. That's way down the line."

"The folks I've just mentioned all believe a fanatical flesh and blood rabbi was killed and then came back to life. They all believe that on Sunday they drink his blood and eat his flesh even though it looks like Welch's Grape Juice and Saltine Crackers, and to a man and woman they believe this dead Jew is going to rise from the grave a second time and save this world from a demonic fiend called the anti-Christ. Are you going to lock them all up in the Northwest Iowa State Hospital with Mr. Schmidt? Why, there wouldn't be enough people in Madisonville to fill the seats in the gallery in this courtroom if you did. What about it, Doctor?"

"You make a good case," said the doctor, "that widespread human beliefs and even belief systems have elements that qualify them as rationally, if not mentally, impaired. But if that were the sole criterion for mental incapacity, then it is quite possible that we'd all qualify for a bunk at the State Hospital. I came in from the parking lot today and consciously stepped over a crack reminding myself of the childhood rhyme 'step on a crack and you break your mother's back' – and my mother has been dead for thirty-five years."

"No, Mr. Lamonte, I don't believe objective rationality is or can be the criterion of evaluating mental illness. The only criterion that makes sense to me as a mental health professional is that of the translation, or possible translation, of those beliefs into action that harms oneself or other humans one comes in contact with. Belief in Santa Claus is harmless enough, even belief in an evil personification of Santa Claus. However, assaulting or killing every man with a white beard one sees on a mission to eliminate the evil Santa Claus threat from the world is a different matter. Killing yourself because you have become the evil Santa Claus is a different matter."

"What about Mr. Schmidt, in your professional opinion Doctor, makes him such a threat to himself or others as to warrant involuntary commitment?" Mr. Lamonte asked.

"Can I see the record?" Doctor Feingold asked.

"Sure," said Mr. Lamonte taking the record from the Bailiff and handing it to Dr. Feingold.

Thumbing through the pages of the file, Dr. Feingold said, "In answer to the question if God instructed you to kill your sons, your wife, or even yourself, would you carry out those instructions? Mr. Schmidt answered 'I don't know, I guess I'd have to.' He rattled off several incoherent phrases in front of the night admissions nurse at the State Hospital in tears. He told my colleague at the State Hospital that the most important person in the universe believed he wasn't crazy, but he declined to elaborate on who that most important person was. I suspect the most important person Mr. Schmidt believes in is the same voice who dictated to him his latest book, or so he attests in the forward to the book."

Dr. Feingold produced the copy of Tom's book that he had been given by Sueann out of a briefcase on the floor at the doctor's feet.

"The book!" Tom shouted out from his seat at the table next to Mr. Lamonte. "Oh Sueann," he said dejectedly. "You gave them the book?"

"Your Honor," protested Ms. Minden rising to her feet.

"Sit down, Ms. Minden," the Judge said. "And you too, Mr. Lamonte. This is an informal proceeding under the Code of Practice. Mr. Schmidt, come on up here, Sir, and talk to me a minute."

Tom got up and walked up to the front of the Judge's bench.

"Tell me about your book over there," the Judge said.

"Well Judge, dadgumit," said Tom, "that's my book. My private papers, and it contains my innermost thoughts and prayers and hopes. It's private, that's all. It's just not right that something as private and intimate as that would be given out and put on display in a courtroom and thrown back into my face to prove something."

"Who did you give the book to, Mr. Schmidt?" asked the Judge.

"Sueann, Your Honor," replied Tom. "My wife, but just to her and only because she demanded to see it, not so she could hand it over to other people and make fun of me."

"Well, Mr. Schmidt," said the Judge, "you can go back over there and sit down with your lawyer. Counsel, I happen to agree with Mr. Schmidt with regard to the privacy of his personal papers he refers to as his 'book'."

"Your Honor, can I be heard on this point?" said Ms. Minden rising from her chair.

"No, you can't, Ms. Minden. I've already ruled on the issue, and I don't want to hear anything more about it. You can take the book from Dr. Feingold and give it back to Mr. Schmidt right now. I'm not going to hear any evidence on this so-called book. Now Mr. Lamonte, do you have anything further on cross-examination?"

"No, Your Honor," said Mr. Lamonte.

"Call your next witness, Ms. Minden," the Judge said.

"Your Honor, in connection with the doctor's testimony we would offer, introduce and file into evidence the entire hospital record regarding Mr. Schmidt, and with that sole evidentiary offering, rest," said Ms. Minden as the doctor left the witness stand and resumed his chair at the counsel table.

"O.K. Mr. Lamonte," said the Judge. "Your turn. What do you have?"

"Judge, I would like to call Reverend Dykes to the stand."

"Wait just a minute," said the Judge. "Mr. Lamonte, what is this good man of the cloth going to add to my understanding of the facts in this case?"

"Judge," said Mr. Lamonte, "Reverend Dykes is Mr. Schmidt's pastor and is prepared to testify as to the beliefs and practices of the Church in the Fields where Mr. Schmidt worships."

"How is that an issue in this case, counselor?" asked the Judge. "My wife reads the horoscope to me every morning over coffee. I don't believe a word of it, but that does not make her factually or legally mentally impaired as far as the court is concerned. Does he have anything else to say?"

"Well, Your Honor, as Mr. Schmidt's pastor, Reverend Dykes will testify that on several occasions when he spoke to Mr. Schmidt . . ."

"Wait a minute!" the Judge called out. "You're not going to call Reverend Dykes to the stand to talk about what Mr. Schmidt here has told him in months and years past – waiving the priest-penitent privilege – and then keep Mr. Schmidt himself off the stand. That's not going to happen in my courtroom. If you think Mr. Schmidt has something valuable to say, put him on the stand. But a preacher is not going to tell me what a man told him with the man sitting in my courtroom available to testify himself. Got that?"

"Yes, Your Honor," said Mr. Lamonte. "I suppose with Your Honor's ruling we have no witnesses to call. The defense rests as well."

"I want to testify," said Tom standing up. "Judge, I've been locked up and haven't seen my family for three days. Do I have a right to say something?"

"Your Honor, the defense is *not* calling Mr. Schmidt to the stand," said Mr. Lamonte.

"Your objection is noted," said the Judge. "Let the record reflect that the court is calling Mr. Schmidt to the stand who poses no personal objection to testifying. Mr. Schmidt, come on up here, sir, and stand there while the Bailiff swears you in."

Mr. Lamonte threw up his hands in disgust and sat down in his chair.

"What do you want to tell me, son?" the Judge asked Tom after he was seated in the witness chair. "Go ahead, don't be shy."

"Judge, Judge, this is a nightmare for me," Tom began. "I'm not cray, Judge. I'm not a threat to my family or anyone else for that matter. All my life people have told me what to do – what I should do – where to go, what university to attend, what jobs to apply for, even who to marry. Maybe I'm a misfit. I don't understand the world. I never have felt that I fit in. If I could just push my beliefs to the side for a moment and look at myself objectively and psychologically, I'd have to say that when I started going to the Church in the Fields I felt for the first time in my life that *this* was something that was really me. Something that I wanted to do. Something that I felt fulfilled in doing. I didn't even want to tell my wife because I knew she'd object to it. She always objects to something or other when it's my idea. I don't know if I even believe in God. I just want to believe in myself. Have my own thoughts. Have my own mind for a change. I wouldn't hurt a fly, Judge. I was an anti-war protestor vegetarian in the '60s. I just want to be left alone, really. I would just like everybody to leave me alone." Tom began to sob. The Judge reached beside him and handed down a box of Kleenex to Tom.

"Any questions, counsel?" the Judge asked. "Ms. Minden? Mr. Lamonte?"

"You can go back over there and sit down by your lawyer," the judge told Tom.

"Counsel, do I gather that neither of you has anything further by way of evidence to present?" the Judge asked. Neither lawyer had any further evidence.

"I do have a few follow-up questions for Dr. Feingold," said the Judge. "You can resume your seat, Doctor," he added. "This is an informal hearing. Doctor Feingold, this isn't your and my first rodeo, so to speak. And I didn't bring my copy of the DSM-III with me today. What are we looking at, Section 290?"

"295-90 Your Honor," said the doctor from his seat at counsel table. "Non-specific or disorganized schizophrenia with or without paranoia."

"I assume this is without evidence of paranoia," said the Judge. "I wouldn't characterize what he just said as paranoia."

"No, Your Honor," said the doctor. "I would agree with you."

"Do you have your DSM-III with you?" the Judge asked.

"Yes, Your Honor," said the doctor.

"Why don't you hand it up to me," said the Judge. "Give it to the Bailiff there."

After a few minutes, the Judge said, "The trouble I have, Doctor, is your working diagnosis of schizophrenia, and I haven't heard any evidence of hallucinations. I'll give you the rest of the positive and negative symptoms. But you're asking me to involuntarily commit a patient on a diagnosis of schizophrenia without evidence of hallucinations. That's kind of a ham on rye without the ham."

"But Your Honor," replied the doctor, "in his book . . ."

"I don't want to hear about the book," the Judge interrupted. "God knows what would have happened if my diary from my teenage years had been discovered by my ex-wife. I'd still be locked up at Northwest. But I'm troubled about this lack of hallucinations. I really am."

"Judge, you may be right," said Dr. Feingold. "Our basic problem is the patient's lack of co-operation. I offered him tests and medication on an outpatient basis. He refused. He is very uncooperative. There is evidence of subterfuge on the patient's part. There is evidence of avolition even in mid-questioning by physicians. If we just had a chance to settle him down a bit and get some co-operation."

"What do you have him on?" the Judge asked.

"Chlorpromazine at first," said the doctor.

"For crying out loud, don't you people ever learn!" the Judge said.

"But we switched that, Your Honor, to haloperidol by injection with orders to substitute medication by mouth when compliant, and he's doing fine," said the doctor.

"We just need some time," added the doctor.

"I don't like it," said the Judge, "but I guess if we went against the flow here and Mr. Schmidt took the righteous spear of Phineas and killed his adulterous neighbor in the next few months we'd all be sitting at the defense table over there next year explaining why we didn't do something to prevent it."

"But Your Honor," said Mr. Lamonte, rising to his feet.

"My problem with your position, Mr. Lamonte," said the Judge interrupting, "has to do with evidence of the Professor Wiggamore courtroom variety. 43,750 people in this county may very well agree with your fundamental defense in this case. In fact, I myself find myself leaning in your client's direction. But on the other hand, this is a court of law and not a Nineteenth Century Camp Meeting in the woods outside of town. A court of law requires evidence and qualified witnesses. The court is faced with your arguments, however persuasive, on the one hand and testimony from a qualified expert witness in the field of mental health on the other. If your client is a simple Christian seeking to find his own path in the complex world, where is a psychologist or psychiatrist to say that under oath? Your constitutional arguments don't get past first base without evidence as to social versus psychiatric norms. Deeds, counsel. Deeds, and not just high-powered words. That comes straight out of the Letter of James in the Bible. Anything more, Mr. Lamonte? Ms. Minden? Then the court is ready to make a ruling. You can all be seated."

"This case came on for hearing pursuant to an expedited assignment on a Chapter 229 Hearing for Involuntary Hospitalization," stated the Judge formally. "Ms. Nora Minden for the County. Mr. Clifton Lamonte for the defense. Upon hearing the evidence and examining the countenance and demeanor of the defendant firsthand, the court is of the opinion that the patient in protective custody, Mr. Thomas Schmidt, currently suffers from a serious mental impairment that both predisposes him to self-injury or the substantial certainty of injury to others as well as prevents him from caring for his own needs. Accordingly, the court hereby remands Mr. Schmidt to the Northwest Iowa State Hospital for a complete psychiatric evaluation and interim care regimen as it sees fit to protect both the patient and the public, which the court additionally finds to be the least restrictive form of treatment under the circumstances. The State Department of Hospitals is hereby ordered to submit a complete evaluation to the court for further review not more than 180 days from this order. Ms. Minden, will you prepare a formal order and circulate it to your opponent for approval?"

"Yes, Your Honor," said Ms. Minden, rising.

The Judge rose and walked through the side door to his right as the Bailiff announced in a loud voice, "court is adjourned until 9 a.m. tomorrow morning." The gallery was astir with people talking and moving around.

"Come on," said Nick suddenly beside Tom. "Let's get out of here."

"Back to the hospital?" Tom asked.

"Yeah, I'm afraid so, Tom," said Nick hugging Tom with a strong right hand. "It's gonna be O.K."

Chapter Twenty-One

The Northwest Iowa State Hospital, formerly the Western Iowa Lunatic Asylum, was built in 1897 and was one of the last of the so-called Kirkbride Plan Asylums popular in the Nineteenth Century. Philadelphia psychiatrist Thomas Kirkbride, a social reformer in the much needed area of kind treatment to the mentally impaired, had formulated a theory that mental illness was a disease, and – like any other disease known at the time encumbering patients – could be relieved or at least lessened by sunlight, fresh air and a modicum of patient recuperative isolation. Accordingly, Kirkbride Asylums tended to have high ceilings, long airy corridors, large patient rooms and plenty of large windows. The grounds of these hospitals tended to be extensive as well and not infrequently included working farms and pastures. The believed curative benefit of these institutions was never completely tested before it became quite evident in both the United States and abroad that the expense of upkeep alone would make such institutions impractical to manage on a typical hospital budget.

The four large wings of the Northwest Iowa State Hospital, renamed in 1953 to drop the stigma in the terms of both "lunatic" and "asylum", had an official capacity of nine hundred beds, but in practice the hospital patient population usually was kept at about two hundred fifty-five. Each of the wings A-Alpha, D-Delta and E-Echo were generally filled to capacity at seventy-five beds each divided more or less equally between two corridors, with the B-Bravo Wing being dedicated to a thirty-bed admission and evaluation ward. Unlike the days of the 1920's and 1930's, hospital patients were no longer compelled – or even allowed – to work in the chicken houses, barns, hog pens and fields comprising much of the hospital's six-hundred forty acre campus, and these once picturesque outbuildings, fences and silos now sat in utter ruin and abandonment. The Iowa State Department of Hospitals did, however, lease out six-hundred acres of the property to Hayes County farmers for corn production which had the effect in the summer and fall months of making the gothic-appearing hospital to rather seem like a red brick island or giant brick ship sitting amidst the swells of a veritable ocean of green – crisscrossed only by the black tarmac of Iowa State Highway 67 and the interstate highway in the distance which one could see from the third story rooms.

Adjacent to the main hospital building was an abandoned yellow brick two-story edifice with an almost inexplicable flat roof for this area of Iowa. This building, with its rusted metallic window fixtures, double front etched glass doors, and overgrown hedges, was the former Hospital Clinic where from 1936 to 1949 various psychiatric medical procedures were performed on patients at the hospital. Some of the procedures performed at the clinic were of the cutting-edge variety, including the administration of insulin shock and electro-convulsive therapies, and from 1939 to 1946 the performance of three hundred fifty-seven pre-frontal lobotomies.

Almost all of the lobotomies were performed with instruments fashioned or invented by Dr. Walter Freeman – an early advocate of the procedure. Indeed, in April, 1946, Dr. Freeman had visited the clinic in his customized "lobotomobile" van and had demonstrated his newly invented "leucotome" instrument to hospital and clinic staff by performing a pre-frontal transorbital lobotomy without anesthesia on Ms. Andrea Stevens Whitcombe, a retired high school teacher from Madisonville and a patient of the hospital at the time with a diagnosis of "unrelenting depression."

When Tom was returned to the hospital following his court appearance, he was rather surprised when Nick drove the hospital van past the B-Bravo Wing delivery entrance and proceeded on to the mid-wing entrance of another extensive part of the hospital he subsequently learned was the E-Echo Wing. Nick produced a key from a large ring on a chain attached to his belt and opened the wire reinforced glass double doors. Sammy walked Tom down a short hall to a nurse's station. Like the nurse's station he had seen on the B-Bravo Wing, a greenish ceramic tile covered the centrally located enclave, above which extended desk-level to ceiling plate glass. A woman dressed in pale blue hospital scrubs sat behind the desk area just to the rear of an opening in the glass, and behind her three or four others either sat or stood at the open fronted file cabinets.

"Schmidt, Thomas A.," Sammy said smiling to the nurse.

"We'll take him from here, flat foot," the woman said smiling as she rose from her chair and walked around the partition.

"If this old hag causes you any trouble, just glare and hiss at her for me," Sammy said laughing as he shook Tom's hand. "You're in good hands, Tom," he added. "Good luck to you."

"Yeah, before you know it, Sammy and I will be coming to get you to drive you home," said Nick as he also shook Tom's hand.

"We were just talking about you," said the nurse to Tom. "We just saw you on the Five O'clock News in the lounge – well, not *you* exactly but a bunch of people on the steps of the courthouse rallying in support of you. Anyway, that's what the news guy said."

"It was on the news?" asked Tom in a concerned voice.

"Yeah, but you can see it again when they re-play it on the ten o'clock segment," said the nurse. "It must be very nice to have so many friends and well-wishers. I can tell you it makes all the difference in the world to have a strong support network in shortening hospital stays. All the difference. Now, I asked for your things from the admit ward, but they said you didn't have anything.

Somebody did drop off a suitcase for you sometime today that the front office sent over, and someone else from the university delivered your mail – at least it looks like mail in a big yellow envelope. Anyway, I got Tina to put everything in your room. Tina is one of the nursing aides that works this corridor on days, and I'm Ethel Mae. I guess you can tell that by the name tag. Oh well, let's get you settled."

Tom followed the nurse up a flight of stairs to the second floor and down a long corridor toward a bright sun-lit lounge at the end full of large windows without curtains or blinds. Stopping briefly at a large door with a small square window, Ethel Mae pushed the door open with her left hand. "This is our dayroom," said the nurse. "There are a bunch of games in that cabinet under the window. The television is currently on the blink, but it's supposed to be fixed this week. We have a few books – not many actually, just a set of encyclopedias, some Gideon Bibles and books the Salvation Army dropped off."

At the large wooden table in the middle of the room an older man sat over a checkerboard with pieces on it, but no opponent was in the immediate vicinity. A very thin middle-aged woman stood by the windows on the far side of the room holding a green metallic ashtray in the upturned palm of her left hand, smoking. Neither person acknowledged the appearance of Tom and the nurse even to the point of looking up. A dirty tin colored thirty-cup coffee urn sat on a table in the corner with three stacks of styrofoam cups to its side. Multiple cylindrical boxes of sugar and creamer flanked the urn's other side, and numerous used red stir sticks lay in the midst of white grainy spills on the table.

"You can come here any time you want that you're not in session," Ethel Mae said releasing the dayroom door to close on its own and continuing to walk briskly down the hall. "Down at the end is the sunroom which gives you a good view – if you like corn that is. You can smoke in the sunroom area and the dayroom, but not in your room or the room of another patient. All smoking is supervised."

Ethel Mae stopped at room E-212, some twenty feet short of the sunroom, and held the door open for Tom to enter. "And here we are!" the nurse said exuberantly turning on the room's garish overhead fluorescent light. Except for the fact that this room had two metal casement windows, it was nearly identical to what Tom's accommodations had been on the B-Bravo Wing. The bed opposing Tom's was made up, but no one was present.

"For the time being you don't have a roommate," Ethel Mae said. "There's no telling around here, though, when you'll get one."

On his bed Tom saw his small gray Samsonite suitcase from home upon which sat his bed slippers, and next to the suitcase was a large yellow University Mail envelope. As soon as the nurse had excused herself, Tom sat on his bed and picked up the envelope. Inside was half a dozen department and college fliers announcing student deadlines or upcoming events, but Tom's attention immediately fell upon a white business-sized envelope with a return address of the Chancellor's Office. Tearing the envelope open he withdrew a single page letter. The letter read:

Dear Associate Professor Schmidt,
    It was with deep concern that I heard about your medical

situation, and please know that the heart-felt best wishes and prayers of the entire university community go out to you and your family during what we all hope will be a short and productive recuperation period. I have formally placed you on administrative leave pending further information about your condition. I want you to be reassured that provisions have been made to hire a contract instructor to conduct your classes and examinations for the entire balance of this semester, if necessary, and that everything is in order. I personally hope you will be able to resume your teaching responsibilities at least by September 5 of this year when the next regularly scheduled semester begins. However, it is also my administrative duty to remind you of the rather blunt and unforgiving wording of Section 532(b) of the University Health & Retirement Policy:

However, any non-tenured contract instructor or associate professor not returning to his or her customary post after being placed on administrative leave for 120 consecutive days or at the beginning of the next regularly scheduled fall or spring semester, whichever occurrence is first, shall be struck from the University's active teaching rolls.

All the very best, and may God bless,
Homer Post, Chancellor

"What's that, a Dear John letter?" a voice said from across the room. Tom looked up to see a man with graying hair, neatly creased tweed trousers, house slippers with argyle socks, and a turtleneck sweater seated on the bed opposite him.

"Basically," Tom said. "God bless you. Drop dead. We're going to fire you."

"Ralph Simionedes," the man said rising and leaning over to shake Tom's hand. "I guess we have been assigned the same jail cell."

"The nurse said I didn't have a roommate," answered Tom.

"Arrogant so-and-so," the man replied. "Anything to negate my existence. Maybe one of these days I'll negate my own existence just to spite them."

"Have you been here long?" Tom asked.

"Seventeen years off and on – mostly on," replied Ralph.

"Seventeen years!" Tom exclaimed in dismay. "Seventeen years?"

"The so-and-sos who govern the E-Echo Wing are laboring under two serious delusions," said Ralph, "the first one being that we are all – to a man and woman – suffering from a disease they have created and named schizophrenia, and the second one being that this mythical disease has a mythical cure. All one has to do is remove the symptoms of the mythical disease and there is a mythical cure of it."

"The psychiatrist in court said he had diagnosed me with schizophrenia," replied Tom.

"That's what we were all diagnosed with on this floor – and half of the next one up – on E-Echo Wing," said Ralph. "It's a neat little 'File 13' to label people with when the establishment – that's them – can't figure out why talented, educated and insightful people – that's us – don't fit into their prefabricated, jet mold world. We're schizophrenics. We're freaks. We're just plain nuts."

"They have a way of punishing you for your world view," replied Tom, "and your friends . . ."

"*Especially* your friends," interrupted Ralph.

"How did you come to get in here in the first place?" Tom asked.

"Well, I taught classics at the University of Athens for fifteen years," began Ralph.

"A university professor!" Tom exclaimed.

"No, no, not really that distinguished," replied Ralph. "I grew up in a Greek-American family in Davenport. Greek Orthodox Church, the whole bit. In 1956 with a master's degree in Ancient Greek and Latin I couldn't find a teaching job – or any other job for that matter unless I lied about my education and picked up a shovel. Anyway, one Sunday I saw an ad in the *Chicago Tribune* for anyone looking for a teaching job overseas. I wrote to the post office box, started a dialogue – they found out I could speak Greek – and two months later I was on a ship bound for the Mediterranean and the land of the ancients. The Greeks were gracious – everyone in the teaching profession there is respectfully called 'professor' from kindergarten on up – but the pay was lousy. I barely made ends meet in a slum apartment in Piraeus. But I got to travel in between teaching sessions, and I went to the islands and Turkey and once to Egypt."

"That's a long way away from here," said Tom.

"Yeah, I know," said Ralph. "And I should have stayed in Greece. But I came home from time to time to visit my parents, and then when they were gone, to see my brother in Des Moines."

"And so?" Tom asked.

"It was probably the Helios thing," said Ralph. "In fact, it *was* the Helios thing, but I didn't catch on at first. I honestly, truly – and naively as it turned out – thought Roy was interested in the revelations about Helios that I had uncovered, especially in my multiple visits to the Island of Rhodes. It had become somewhat of a passion with me. After a while every chance I got I took the overnight ferry from Piraeus to Rhodes. Ahhh, I wish I were there now. I could only afford to stay in the old city, but that's actually where I wanted to be – mosquitoes, dead cats, fish market, ruins, junk shops and all. My first visit was just by way of curiosity. I was a tourist, albeit one who could read Attic Greek. I should have been suspicious. I should have been suspicious the first evening when I watched the sun disappear in a giant red ball over the mountains of Symi. Oh Helios! How magnificent! It took my breath away. And then the next morning to see the sun rise in a shower of gold over the hills of Turkey across the water. It was awe-inspiring, my friend. Ah, my friend . . . ?"

"Tom," Tom Schmidt responded. "Tom Schmidt."

"Well, it was awe-inspiring, friend Tom," said Ralph. "Simply awe-inspiring. But then on the afternoon of the second day on that first trip, as I was rummaging in a rotten wooden box in an old shop off the market thoroughfare by the Turkish Baths, I found it."

"Found what?" asked Tom

"The seal. The seal of Helios – the Great and Eternal God Helios. The Sun God, man. The sun itself, and the source of all energy. Oh, the ancient clay seal was broken to be sure, friend Tom. Just a part of the golden chariot of Helios was there, and only one of the horses' heads on the front. On the back was a depiction of Helios rising over Symi – just as I had seen, but only half of the Symi Mountain Range was shown on the fragment. But the inscription, friend Tom. The inscription! In perfect

Attic Greek on the front were the words 'Forever Helios has risen and will ever rise', and on the back the verse continued 'to ever, ever warm the earth and skies.' Our god Helios!" Ralph exhaled audibly as he fell back onto his bed.

"And?" asked Tom.

"And – well, and this seal answered everything as far as I was concerned," said Ralph sitting up again. "Everything! It answered questions that had not yet even formed in my mind then. I had read the classics – we all have. And I had read Pindar – we all have. *Praise the sea maid, daughter of Aphrodite, bride of Helios, this Isle of Rhodes!* I knew that the Island of Rhodes was sacred to Helios. Excuse me for stating the obvious, but what we didn't know! What I didn't know. Phoebus the shining orb. Helios Panoptes, the *All Seeing*. Hyperion of Homer. The inspiration of the Great Colossus of Rhodes. The focal point of the Corinthian Temple to Apollo. And even before that, as Viracocha, the inspiration for Tiwanaku in South America. And even before that the great city of Heliopolis in Egypt. And even more before that the great and enigmatic Sphinx in witness to the all-consuming greatness of Helios in eleven thousand years B.C."

"And after all of that?" asked Tom.

"Why dear friend Tom," replied Ralph. "After that *everything*. Simply *everything* mankind knows of the godhead is Helios inspired. Take the god of the Hebrews: 'the Lord God is a sun and a shield,' said the Psalmist. 'The sun of righteousness shall arise with healing,' said the Prophet Malachi. The flame and 'Divine Luster' of the Zoroastrians. It is all the same. *He* is all the same. 'The true light which lighteth every man that cometh into the world,' proclaimed John the Evangelist. The Uncreated Light of the Desert Fathers . . ."

"You know the Desert Fathers?" interrupted Tom, aghast.

"Well, of course, friend Tom," replied Ralph. "We have all read about them. But the point is that all personifications of the godhead are a part of the One True Light. Call it the sun. Call it Amun Ra as the Egyptians did. Call it Helios or Hyperion or Apollo as the eastern ancients did. Call it Viracocha as the western ancients did. Call it Jehovah, Jesus, or the Uncreated Light. It is all the same. *He* is all the same. He is the One True Light of the world upon which we all depend from moment to moment and without which we would all perish, and rather quickly. At dawn and all through the day the loving fingers of Helios strokes the earth as a harpist lovingly strokes the strings of an instrument, and the celestial music of Helios is our all in all."

"I'd like to see the seal of Helios," said Tom.

"Alas," replied Ralph. "My brother Roy asked for the seal – supposedly to study it – and I never saw it again. Every time I've asked for it, he has pretended it doesn't exist. My notes are gone too, and my journal. My journal was probably the real reason I was sent here the first time. I shouldn't have written down some of the things I did in English. Now, I only have my memories of Rhodes and the dawn in the sunroom down the hall. We can't see the setting of the sun from this wing."

Nurse Ethel Mae poked her head through the doorway. "Mr. Schmidt, they've just started serving in the wing cafeteria," she announced. "You must be famished after yesterday. Why don't you come along with me and I'll show you the ropes?"

Tom rose from his bed. "Are you coming?" he asked Ralph.

"Yeah, I'll go with you," said the nurse. "Come on."

"Naw," said Ralph. "These so-and-sos pretty much ignore me around here and I pretty much ignore them. I'll get something later."

Chapter Twenty-Two

When Tom returned to room 212 after eating, Ralph Simionedes was nowhere to be seen, and so after sticking his still packed Samsonite suitcase into the wardrobe nearest his bed and putting the university mail into the drawer in the side table, Tom walked out into the hall and down to the sunroom. The sunroom itself was less of a room and more of an extended space at the end of the hallway. There was a green naugahyde seating arrangement with an upholstered sofa and matching chairs in front of the hall-wide series of windows. Next to one chair was a standing cigarette ash tray with two facing silver tone flamingos presiding over the butts and half-burnt matches. The sun had gone down behind – or actually *in front of* the hospital – and the long shadow of the building extended eastward over the rear lawn for thirty yards or so until the beginning of the cornfields. The corn was dark green in the declining light and seemingly stretched to the horizon as far as Tom could see. From the sunroom window Tom could not see the entrance drive to the hospital, but just at the edge of his field of vision to his far left he could see what part of the hospital cemetery must be. Just past the corner of the cemetery Tom could see – and stretching all across his vista to the right – the nearly black Highway 67 and its ditches as it cut through the cornfields between the hospital grounds and the vast tracks of fields further to the east.

On the far side of the highway nearly opposite him, Tom could see a billboard rising from the cornfield. It faced south-bound traffic and was illuminated at night by three equally spaced spotlights fastened to the top of the sign. It read:

Hayes County Corn Growers Can Count on Super Yields Using ISAI 48 – 10

**Available Through Your County Agent
Iowa State Agricultural Institute
Iowa State University**

Tom sat in one of the chairs for a long time looking at the fields grow progressively darker until the illuminated billboard commanded his entire attention. He wondered what ISAI 48-10 was. Hybrid seed of some kind? Fertilizer? He didn't have a clue. When Tom returned to room 212 Ralph Simionedes had still not appeared. He closed the door, turned out the light, undressed and slipped into bed – completely and utterly alone and without a plan as to what to do. In the course of one day he had lost his chance for an early release from this prison – no, in some ways it was worse than a prison – he had become totally alienated from his wife of twelve years, and it looked as if he would lose his job at the university. How could Sueann have done such a thing to him? And what about the boys? He hadn't seen them now in – what – three days? More than three days, really, he thought to himself. This was a total nightmare.

The only way Tom could keep his composure was to not think about everything that was happening or the implications of what was happening. He would tackle things as they presented themselves and concentrate on just getting out of the hospital. The Judge had said a report was due in 180 days. Tom wondered if that necessarily meant he had to stay in the hospital for that long. He would explain his situation to the doctor when he saw him next. He would cooperate with that quack and see if he couldn't work the system for a release. Anything, just to get out of here.

"Knock, knock!" a cheerful voice rang out. The door opened a few feet and the head of a woman poked through. "I didn't realize you were down already," the woman said. "I'm the night nurse on this wing. I need to bring you your meds before you go to sleep, and Ethel Mae said you might be interested in seeing the ten o'clock news tonight. The television set in the day room isn't working, but you can watch at our set at the nurse's station if you like."

"Why not?" said Tom as he began to throw back the covers and then stopped short.

"Where's your robe and slippers?" the night nurse asked. "They should have had some laid out for you with the toiletries. I'll go get you some. I'll be right back with your meds and the robe," she said disappearing behind the door.

Later, on the little six-inch television screen in the nurse's lounge behind the corridor station Tom watched in his hospital robe and slippers as the camera zoomed in on Reverend Dykes standing on the courthouse steps. In the end, the television coverage was not as bad as Tom had imagined. He listened carefully, and his name was not mentioned once, although for a fleeting instant the camera caught the hospital van with Nick in the driver's seat and Tom with his ear pressed against the back window. In an interview following the court hearing Reverend Dykes was asked by the television reporter whether the church's lawyer would appeal the ruling of Judge Giddeon.

"No, Sir," said Reverend Dykes. "We will not appeal the ruling – at least not in a court of secular law. We have forcefully and persuasively made our point in the cause of religious freedom before Judge Giddeon here today. However, with prayers and supplications we do intend on appealing the matter to the Lord God who is the supreme justice of all the earth. If it is the will of the Lord God that our suffering brother be released from the terrible bonds that confine him, then we will see him again – possibly this Saturday at the Church in the Fields at 10 a.m. out at the Green Wave-Clinton crossroads north of Madisonville. We worship and rest on the 7th day of the week as the Lord God has commanded, and we have a fully staffed nursery for the little ones."

The next morning Tom was amazed not to see Ralph Simionedes in the room or any sign that he had been there. His bed had not been slept in. Tom pulled his Samsonite suitcase out of the wardrobe and opened it. Inside was the pair of pajamas he had received for Christmas the year before, his bulky woolen blue sweater, three pairs of clean underwear, two pairs of white socks, a comb, his worn out toothbrush in a white plastic travel container, and his safety razor without any blades in it. Fastened to the top of the sweater with a piece of scotch tape was a note from Sueann. It read:

Dearest Tom,

I don't know what to say so I guess I'll keep this note brief. I am so sorry about your condition and the doctor having to put you in the State Hospital. I don't want the boys to see you in that terrible place, so for now I am telling them that you had to go out of town to do some school research. I will come see you when I can get up the emotional strength to do so – so bear with me for a little while. You are so changed, and I am having to carry the entire family emotionally all by myself right now. Please try and see things from where I am at. Get well. See you soon.

Love, Sueann

"*Another* Dear John?" came a voice from the other bed. Tom looked up to see Ralph Simionedes sitting on the edge of the bed opposite him.

"Pretty close," said Tom. "She's not ready to come see me, and she's not telling my sons where I am or how I got into this godforsaken place."

"God hasn't forsaken you, Tom," Ralph said, "even if that preacher friend of yours has."

"Oh," said Tom. "I guess you saw the television spot on the news yesterday."

"Pretty pitiful," replied Ralph. "Not you – the preacher's performance."

"Yeah, I guess you get what you pay for," mused Tom out loud.

"Where have you been?" asked Tom. "Were you here at all last night?"

"Oh, I was around," said Ralph. "Near dawn I pray to the rising Helios."

"Does Helios ever answer you?" asked Tom.

"Helios *used to answer me*, and in Attic Greek no less," said Ralph, "but with the Thorazine and the Haldol and the Stelazine and the Mellaril and the Prolixin and Helios only knows what else, it has become very difficult for me to hear the Attic Greek any more. That's what they want, you know. They want you to think the Great Other has gone away just because they pump so many drugs in you that you can't hear the Other's voice. But the Other is still there."

"How do you know, Professor?" asked Tom.

"Ralph," said Simionedes. "Call me Ralph. I'm not really a professor. They just called me that in Greece."

"O.K., Ralph," said Tom. "How do you know that the Great Other – the one Other in the universe that you trust in and you know has faith in you . . . is still there? Is still listening, and still has faith in you?"

"There are ways," replied Ralph. "There are ways. These drugs affect the hearing. They are aimed at eliminating auditory hallucinations and in their broad sweep they often carry many things away with them. But if the Great Other – and let's face it we're both talking about Helios, the Rising Sun, and the Uncreated Light – if the Great Other wants to talk to you then the Other will select a way. Sights, visions, words, phrases on a page. The Other will find a way."

"I know what you mean," said Tom. "He. God that is. The Uncreated Light . . ."

"Helios," interrupted Ralph.

"Yes, Helios," said Tom, "used to speak to me through my computer screen when I found it difficult to hear his voice."

"Signs and wonders, friend Tom," replied Ralph. "Remember signs and wonders. They are the essence of Helios."

After Ralph Simionedes had again declined to join Tom at mealtime, Tom found himself sitting alone at one of the formica-topped tables drinking a cup of black coffee in the wing's dayroom.

"Not eating?" came a voice from a thin woman with stringy brown hair standing beside him. She looked to be in her early thirties and was dressed in jeans without a belt, a white sweatshirt and tennis shoes, although covered up partially with a hospital-issue faded green bathrobe open in the front. Like all hospital-issue robes, the robe's cloth belt was missing. A lit cigarette was pinched between the index finger and thumb of the woman's right hand as if she was holding a dart and was poised to throw it.

"No, not eating," replied Tom. "How can you have an appetite in a place like this?"

"Yeah, it's a dump alright," said the woman. "Mind if I sit down?"

"No," replied Tom. "I don't mind. Have a seat."

"Smoke?" the woman asked producing a package of Newports from her robe pocket and offering the pack to Tom.

"Not since college," said Tom.

"Might as well start again," replied the woman sitting down in the chair opposite Tom. "Everybody in here smokes sooner or later. Coffee and cigarettes – the breakfast of champions."

"Maybe I can get out of here before too long," said Tom.

"By what?" asked the woman, "Playing the game?"

"I was thinking about it," Tom replied. "*Not playing the game* doesn't seem to work."

"Playing the game, not playing the game – it's all the same, and nothing *works*," said the woman waving her dart-like cigarette in the air and punctuating the word 'works' by jabbing the cigarette aggressively toward the dining room door.

"The reason nothing works," she continued, "is that the entire world is not in *working order*. I'm sure you have already noticed that the world – I mean the world *outside there* – is seriously fucked up. If you hadn't, they wouldn't have sent you here. That's our punishment for noticing little things. Like that the world is totally nuts. It's easy to play a little game of cooperation and agree with Silvia or whoever your doctor is . . ."

"Feingold," interrupted Tom. "His name is Feingold."

"What a jerk," the woman commented. Then continuing, she said, "well it's easy to play a little game of cooperation and agree with Feingold that you are crazy – schizophrenic, you name it, but that's not the hard part. What is not so easy is trying to pretend that Feingold's world – that is the world outside in Madisonville, Des Moines, you name it – is *not* crazy. Are you running with me new person? What is your name, anyway? My name is Maggie Mae. Well, my name is *not actually* Maggie Mae. Maggie Mae is my poetic name, my *nom de plume* – you name it."

"What's your real name?" Tom asked.

"That . . . ," the woman said dramatically with a puff on her cigarette. "Damn it, it went out," she complained throwing the butt into the green metallic ashtray on the table. "You know I like these Newports – I mean I really like them. Flavorful, reassuring, aromatic – you name it, but they're not long lived. Like poets, they burn out and burn up just when they are at their peak."

"Zip, Zip," Maggie Mae said around a new cigarette she held clenched in her teeth as she fumbled with a pack of matches.

"Anyway," she continued sucking in a first breath of the now lit cigarette and blowing out the smoke in a long stream to the left of Tom, "my *real name* is for me to know and these yoyos to find out. You know, Dr. Silvia denies this, but it is a fact that somewhere buried under all the dusty code books in Washington D.C. or in the secret caves in the Rockies, or wherever – you name it – there is a Federal law that they can't electroshock you if they don't have your real, actual, *bona fide*, legal name on file."

Maggie Mae half-coughed as she sucked in a big drag of smoke.

"That's *nicotiana tabacum* for you," Tom said adopting a professorial tone. "The American Indians smoked an even stronger kind of tobacco called *nicotiana rustica* that had nine times the nicotine of modern cigarettes and caused serious intoxication, hallucinations and even unconsciousness."

"No shit?" replied Maggie Mae. "I need some of that Injun' tobacco. What brands have it?"

"None today, I'm afraid," said Tom.

"Well, fuck it," she said with resignation.

"You know," said Tom, "I think I'll take a Newport after all." "Now you're talking," replied Maggie Mae pushing the pack

on the table toward Tom.

Tom picked up the box of matches on the table and took out one.

"Turn around," said Maggie Mae.

"Huh?" asked Tom striking the match.

"Turn around and show Mr. Orderly standing over there what you are doing with the match or he'll take 'em away – it's the law around here," Maggie explained.

"Electroshock?" Tom said to Maggie Mae while smiling to the orderly and blowing out his first puff of smoke. "I didn't think they still did that."

"Don't kid yourself," said Maggie Mae. "Have you ever taken a look at those portraits they have hung all down the corridor next to the nurse's station?"

"I don't think I noticed them," replied Tom.

"Well I did," said Maggie Mae, "and I looked them up too in the encyclopedias in the day room. These characters are a gallery of ghouls. Ugo Cerleti, the Italian who invented the electroshock machine. Joseph Meduna, the Hungarian shrink who experimented on patients by inducing so-called *therapeutic* seizures. Manfred Sickle or Sakel, whatever, the Polack shrink who induced insulin shock to treat patients by nearly killing them. There are two or three other ghouls I can't remember right now, but the point is that nothing restrains these people from experimenting on us as the most helpless type of guinea pigs — that is if, and only if, they know your name. By the way new person, what did you say your name was?"

"Tom," Tom said taking in another puff of smoke. "And I'm afraid it's my real name."

"Shit," replied Maggie Mae. "That's bad. Oh, not your name. I think Tom is a perfectly marvelous name. It's just that in here the less *they* know the better. I've got to the point I almost never talk to Dr. Silvia. He just twists things around. I like Kitty the weekend night nurse, but she's kind of fucked up herself. I haven't seen her lately. The rest of the nurses are so upbeat and blasted *professional* I could puke."

"Hey," Maggie Mae said putting out the butt of her cigarette and lighting another Newport, "do you want to hear a poem I wrote?"

"Sure," said Tom putting out the butt remains of his cigarette.

"Want another Newport?" Maggie Mae asked. "You know, I'm close to not being able to think without a Newport. It'll make the poem sound better."

"Well, O.K.," said Tom easing out another Newport from the pack. "You talked me into it."

Maggie Mae pulled a folded piece of paper from her jeans pocket and unwrapped it. Taking a deep drag from her cigarette, she began:

> For the ones who think they can have it their way at
>   McDonalds.
> You're normal.
> For the ones who see the USA in their new Chevrolet.
> You're sane.

For the ones who ask not what their country can do for them.
You're right.
For those who'd walk a mile for a Camel.
You're normal.
For those who wait all year for the Super Bowl.
You're sane.
For those who pray to Jesus and Santa Claus.
You're right.
For those who drink booze without enjoyment.
You're normal.
For those who believe in everybody, even god.
You're sane.
For those who want to help everybody,
  even those who don't need their fucking help.
You're right.
For those who kill so that there will be peace.
You're normal.
For those who say, 'What the hell – let's live it up.'
You're sane.
I'm wrong.
I'm insane.
I'm abnormal.
You are entirely right.

"That's pretty good," said Tom after she had finished. "What's the title of the poem?"

"The public name or the *real* name?" Maggie Mae asked. They both laughed out loud.

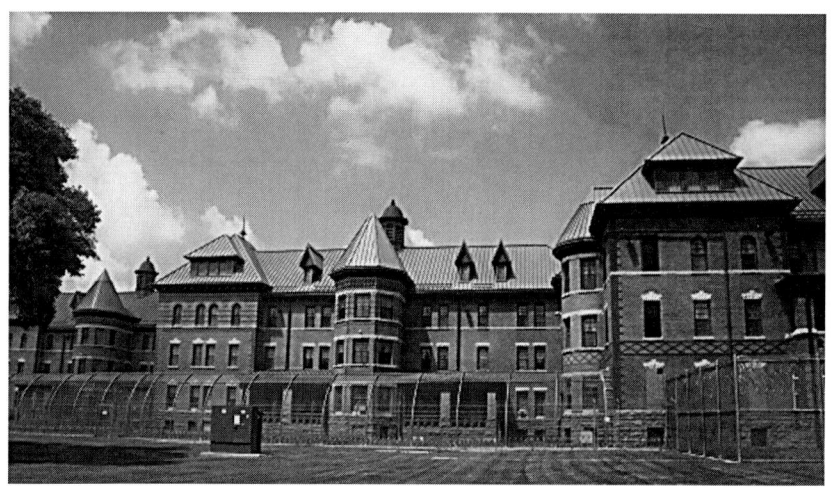

Chapter Twenty-Three

That afternoon Dr. Feingold came to visit on Tom's ward, and Tom was asked to attend a "session" with the doctor in the conference room near the nurse's station.

"Dr. Feingold," said Tom. "I've decided that you have totally won."

"There's no winning or losing in here, Tom," replied the doctor. "We're trying to help you."

"Well, whatever," said Tom. "Just tell me what to do, and I'll do it."

"I'm not so sure it's that easy," replied Dr. Feingold. "We need to get at the root cause of some of the troubles you have been experiencing."

"I may have been *causing* trouble, Doctor," said Tom, "but I do not *feel* troubled."

"Exactly my point," replied Dr. Feingold. "We need to set as at least a preliminary goal your recognition that the behavior you have exhibited is not socially standard. Do you feel your actions in the past few months have been "normal" – well, let's use that word although I usually don't use it and it may not be all that helpful. So, *normal* in contrast to your life before you began to take an intense interest in religion?"

"I guess that depends on what one considers to be normal," replied Tom. "I don't think it is abnormal for a man to believe in God."

"Yes," replied the doctor, "but what kind of god? In the Judeo-Christian traditions man is said to have been made in God's *image* or *likeness*. What do you think God's likeness is? Is it a physical likeness?"

"Well," replied Tom, "according to Jesus, God is a Spirit, not a physical being at all, so at least according to Jesus, God's likeness to man is not physical."

"Well, how about morally?" asked Dr. Feingold. "Is man *morally* made in a God's likeness?"

"I certainly hope not," replied Tom.

"I certainly hope not myself," said the doctor. "All around us we see mankind's injustice and cruelty – and maybe you are more knowledgeable about the Bible than I am, but in the Old Testament isn't the Bible's God portrayed as somewhat of a rough character – I mean that God is depicted as directing a fair amount of killing people, including what we might think of as innocent civilians and little children. Is that just the way God is, in your opinion?"

"I don't know, Doctor," replied Tom. "Maybe in some ways God struggles like we struggle, and maybe the entire universe is in process of some kind. Maybe some of the very questions we ask ourselves are the questions *God* wants answered."

"If that were true," said the doctor, "God wouldn't be all that morally perfect, would he? Didn't Jesus say for humans to be 'perfect, even as your Father which is in heaven is perfect'? Do you think God is *perfect* as depicted in the Old Testament of the Bible?"

"I don't know," said Tom.

"I think that is all we need to discuss today, Tom," said Dr. Feingold.

That evening as Tom sat in the sunroom watching the shadows lengthen over the northern lawn of the hospital, he wondered where Ralph Simionedes had disappeared to. Tom thought him a most unusual and mysterious man, although in some ways Ralph seemed very spiritual. What had Ralph said: that "the Other will find a way to communicate if he wants to?"

"Sights, visions, words, phrases on a page. The Other will find a way?"

As Tom watched the sky darken the three exterior lights at the top of the billboard across the street blinked a few times and came on, followed by swarms of moths becoming attracted to the light.

"The Other will find a way," Tom thought to himself.

"The Other will find a way," Tom said to himself again out loud as he stared at the billboard.

Hayes County Corn Growers Can Count on Super Yields
Using ISAI 48 – 10
Available Through Your County Agent
Iowa State Agricultural Institute
Iowa State University

Tom leaped to his feet. "Isaiah Chapter 48, Verse 10!" Tom exclaimed, and he turned and ran down the hallway and into the dayroom. Maggie Mae was standing by one of the windows holding a Newport in her characteristic dart throwing grip.

"Hey Tom," she said as Tom quickly moved across the room to the wooden shelf holding the Gideon Bibles and religious tracts. Ignoring the woman, Tom grabbed one of the editions with both the Old and New Testaments and fanned through the book until he found the Book of Isaiah.

"What's up, brother?" Maggie Mae asked. "Smitten by the Holy Spirit?"

"Something like that Maggie," Tom replied. "Here it is, Isaiah 48, Verse 10:

Behold, I have refined thee, but not with silver;
I have chosen thee in the furnace of affliction.

Tom clutched the open Bible to his chest and slid down into one of the nearby chairs arranged around the room's center table. It was true, Tom thought, the Other will find a way to speak to a human heart. Waves of relief and joy and love and reassurance poured over Tom as tears moistened both of his eyes. "I have chosen thee in the furnace of affliction," Tom repeated out loud.

Maggie Mae came over and put her non-dart throwing hand on Tom's shoulder. Taking a deep drag from her Newport, she exhaled, asking "You all right Tom?"

"Yeah, I'm all right," answered Tom. "I've just discovered something that I should have known all along. Ralph Simionedes helped me to discover it."

"Ralph Simionedes?" Maggie Mae asked.

"Yeah, Ralph Simionedes," replied Tom. "He's been in and out of here for seventeen years. He's my roommate."

"If you say so," Maggie Mae responded. "How about a Newport? It looks to me like you could use one."

"Sure," said Tom. Then, exhaling his first drag on the Newport, he asked, "Maggie, you're a poet. Would you say that this place is poetically akin to a 'furnace of affliction'?"

"Judging by the devils in here and the torments they put us through – yes, I'd say without hesitation that this hole is a furnace of affliction. Perdition itself," Maggie replied.

Tom put out his Newport halfway through the cigarette.

"Can we keep one of these Bibles in our room?" asked Tom.

"I don't think anyone gives a rat's ass what you do with those Bibles," Maggie Mae replied. "When the nut case holy rollers come around, they bring armfuls of them."

"Thanks," Tom said to Maggie Mae without knowing why. He got up from the table and walked slowly to his room. Down the hall he could see far beyond the big plate glass window the billboard lit up in the distance. "I have chosen thee in the furnace of affliction," he repeated out loud.

On Sunday, Tom was uncharacteristically happy and actually joyful to see Father Grey from St. Albans Episcopal Church when he made his rounds on the ward.

"Father Grey," asked Tom, "is God perfect?"

"But of course, he is," the priest replied. "Perfect in every conceivable way."

"Then why is God depicted so ruthlessly in the Old Testament – so sternly?" Tom asked.

"God is perfect," replied the priest. "However, man's perception and appreciation of God is highly imperfect. The Apostle Paul compared our human appreciation of God as looking through a glass darkly – that shades and to some extent distorts the true nature of God. As Christians, we should consider the Holy Scriptures as a whole and *compelling* – without dwelling on the literal meaning of each and every chapter and verse."

"Then God did not literally order the Israelites to kill the native inhabitants of Palestine and take their land because the Jews were the so-called 'favored nation'?" Tom asked.

"I don't know," replied Father Grey. "I can tell you personally, Tom, that as a man and as a Christian I simply can't believe that was true. If I did, they would have to make a permanent place for me in here, because the thought that a universal God existed who would do such a thing would drive me . . ." The priest hesitated.

"Crazy like me?" Tom asked.

"Mad," replied the priest. "Just mad."

That evening, in his room, Tom retrieved "the book" that the Judge had ordered returned to him from his little wardrobe. Opening the book at random he read from the Chapter *Perfect Ecstasy*:

> *Each breath comes now with welcome ecstasy.*
> *My heartbeat song's a melody of love.*
> *We are the earth below and stars above.*
> *We are the autumn leaves, we are the wind.*
> *We are the one who sent, the one who went.*
> *We are Creation in this one moment.*

Remembering fondly of the days and weeks he had listened to the Uncreated Light dictate the book to him, Tom was suddenly happier and more at peace than he had been for some time. He turned the pages until, in *The Songs of Creation* he found the passage:

> *You had no birth and neither will you die.*
> *You are the ancient oak and rocky crag.*
> *You are the rain that fell upon the earth,*
> *You are the moon that bathes the earth with light.*
> *In ecstasy each day and starry night*
> *You are all Creation in mind and sight.*

In an instance of revelation and insight, Tom suddenly understood within his own being that the entire controversy surrounding the Bible and its "truths" was totally and completely irrelevant *to him*. Unlike the Apostle Paul – or at least Father Grey's *understanding* of the Apostle Paul's *understanding* – the nature of God need not be distorted or incomplete. One only need listen to the Uncreated Light as it makes itself known.

Tom missed the voice of the Uncreated Light speaking to him. Of all the voices and sounds in the world – the Uncreated Light represented his most loving comforter, supporter, and teacher. With the voice of the Uncreated Light, Tom had understanding and – most of all – happiness. Without the voice of the Uncreated Light Tom suffered alienation and loneliness. If Ralph Simionedes was right and the medications given in the hospital stifled the voice of God, then there was only one solution to unhappiness of all kinds. Tom would stop taking the pills they gave him. He would have to simulate swallowing them – hide them in his hand or under his tongue – something. They couldn't know he was not taking the medicine, or they would force him to take it. He had seen them force Maggie Mae to take her medication just the other day. He would do anything he had to do in order to get the voice of the Uncreated Light back.

The next session with Dr. Feingold was strained.

"You're trying to get me to not believe in the Uncreated Light, aren't you," Tom said at the outset of the meeting.

"I don't know why this concept of belief has you so upset, Tom," said the doctor. "I totally don't understand this idea of "belief" with either my "intellectual" mind or my "spiritual" mind and despite all I have heard about it from some of my patients. Why would the creator of the universe with infinite mercy and love for all creation possibly *care* whether his own *divinity* was *believed* in by his creation? Is the real God that big of an egomaniac? Does the real God even care if some of his creations are "unbelievers"? I seem to recall Jesus' words quoted in the Gospel of Luke, 'love your enemies, and you shall be the children of the highest, for God is kind unto the unthankful and to the evil.' So, I couldn't care less whether you believe in a god or not – and probably any god that actually exists cares not in the slightest himself, herself, or itself whether you are a believer or not."

"I thought my beliefs were the whole point of keeping me in here," Tom replied somewhat sarcastically.

"The whole *point* of keeping you in here, Tom," replied Dr. Feingold, "is that you have failed to grasp reality, and you live in a fantasy world where you hear voices telling you what to do."

"Welcome to Twentieth Century America," said Tom. "I pledge allegiance to the flag, of the United . . ."

"*Some people*," Dr. Feingold interrupted, "find solace in talking to imaginary friends or in writing about their frustrations in their diaries. Some even talk to their dogs and cats. But, Tom, you call your imaginary friend 'God Almighty', and your friend talks back. The fact that you call your imaginary friend God does not make it any more real than any other imaginary friend of the dog or cat variety, and you must realize that no god is going to swoop down from heaven and rescue you from this place. Oh, you can be rescued, to be sure, but *you* will have to affect that rescue yourself. Only you can make yourself well again."

"Go to hell," said Tom turning to the wall.

"Tom? Tom?" asked Dr. Feingold, but Tom remained immobile and rigid.

"Well," said Dr. Feingold at last. "I guess our session has ended." After several tortured minutes, Dr. Feingold got up and left the conference room.

"Mr. Schmidt is upset," he told a nurse at the station. "Thirty milligrams of Dalmane, p.o. That will help him rest."

Chapter Twenty-Four

"I told youuushuu," said Maggie Mae inhaling a large breath of Newport the next morning over coffee.

"I told you," she repeated exhaling the smoke as she spoke, "that playing the game or not playing the game – it's all the same. Nothing works."

"I'll grant you that," said Tom reaching for the pack of Newports on the stained table top.

"Look," Tom said. "I'm helping myself to your Newports, but I found a ten-dollar bill in the pants pocket I came in here with. I don't know where to buy the damned things, but if you can get us a carton, I'll split them with you."

"Done deal," said Maggie Mae taking the ten-dollar bill. "My brother –in-law's an asshole, but he does keep me in Newports. He shows up every other Sunday, so my sister doesn't have to look me in the eye, be alone with me, suffer guilt – you name it, for putting me in this dump. In the meantime, help yourself. I'm not even low yet."

"Look," Maggie Mae said as Tom lit his Newport. "Do you know what the definition of 'psychotic' is?"

"Huh?" replied Tom as he exhaled a stream of smoke. "Psychotic, crazy – fucked up, you name it. What they have down in both your and my charts as justification for keeping us locked up in here."

"No," replied Tom. "I don't know what the definition of psychotic is – at least not formally speaking."

"Well, it is defined as quote 'out of touch with reality and delusional' unquote," said Maggie Mae. "As in you and I are out of touch with *their* reality."

Tom said nothing as he inhaled the smoke deep into his lungs.

"Look," said Maggie Mae, "I've been researching in the Encyclopedia Britannica in the day room, and these bastards whose pictures are on the wall by the nurse's station are not the only game in town, so to speak."

"What are you talking about?" Tom asked.

"Psychosis, Tom. Schizophrenia, *Tom. Duh*!" she said. "That's you and me to these jerk-offs."

"Proceed, Professor," said Tom taking another puff. "Why are not those bastards on the wall in the hallway the only game in town?"

"Because, my friend", she replied, "of the doctors and shrinks whose portraits are conveniently *not* on the wall by the nurse's station. I wrote some notes – if you don't mind," she said taking a wrinkled and carelessly folded paper from her jeans pocket.

"By all means, consult your notes," said Tom.

"Take Professor Thomas Szasz, author of the book *The Myth of Mental Illness*. Professor Szasz argued that everybody – including you and me – has a right to bodily and mental self-ownership, and the right to be free of interference from others. Look, I wrote down this quote, Tom. The professor said, 'if you talk to God, you are praying; if God talks to you, you have schizophrenia. If the dead talk to you, you are a spiritualist; if you talk to the dead, you are a schizophrenic.' Isn't that cool? I can't wait to hit Silvia with that quote in session."

Tom took a deep drag on his Newport and blew the smoke towards the ceiling.

"Unimpressed, huh?" Maggie Mae said. "Well get a load of this. Professor Szasz wrote that labeling someone as *insane* or a *drug addict* (and baby that's me) is the same as the persecutions used to be for witches, the demon possessed, gypsies and homosexuals. He thought that these types of branded people are scapegoats and society's underclass."

"Get this, Tom," Maggie Mae said leaning over the table to get closer. "One of the ghouls I forgot the name of the other day. His mug shot is there. Right by the session room door. The Josef Mengele of so-called mental illness in the United States. So-called 'Dr.' Walter Freeman, the popularizer of transorbital lobotomies. Zap, zap! Right through the eye socket into the brain with an ice pick. This man was worse than a killer. He left his victims – all forty thousand of them before he was through –

without a conscious mind. Without a conscious soul. Can you believe they let that hypocrite's picture stay up there? Anyway, the great Dr. Freeman is quoted as saying his lobotomies would quote *make good American citizens of society's misfits, schizophrenics* (baby, that's us), *homosexuals and radicals* unquote."

"Jesus H. Christ!" Maggie Mae said snuffing out her Newport butt and taking another cigarette from the now communal packet on the table. "Professor Szasz was so right. We don't think like them. Our reality is not screwed up like theirs is, so they 'fix us' by branding us as schizophrenics and locking up us in this hole. I'm never giving them my real name. Never."

"Well, I don't see how all this is going to help me get out of here," said Tom taking another Newport from the pack without asking and picking up the box of safety matches Maggie Mae had thrown on the table.

"We're never going to get out of here," replied Maggie Mae, "at least not for long. We're tagged. We're marked with the sign of the beast. We can never credibly speak our mind again or have an interesting insight again or go against popular opinion again or root for the underdog in a political race again. We're screwed. Everybody will put on a big shit-eating grin when they are around us and clap like they are affirming a three-year-old even when we mess up. Don't you see? There's a lobotomy a sadistic monster like Freeman can perform and then there's a social lobotomy that is performed when they stamp 'schizophrenic' on your medical record and lock you up in a sewer like this. Actually, Freeman's lobotomies were kinder. When he screwed up your brain you were no longer conscious of the wry smiles – the whispers. When you are socially lobotomized, you're screwed twice over. You are branded a lunatic and you *know* they *know*. Good luck finding a job."

It was a full three days after Tom stopped swallowing the pills the nurses presented in a paper med cup twice a day, that Ralph Simionedes walked into Tom's room right when he was waking up from a nap.

"Ralph, it's great to see you!" exclaimed Tom. "Where have you been?"

"Oh around," said Ralph. "They want to perform some kind of procedure on me, but I won't let them. Even if they force me, I won't let them."

"How is that accomplished, Ralph?" Tom asked. We're locked up in here and there's nowhere to go."

"There's *always* somewhere to go Tom," said Ralph. "Not all people have the courage and fortitude to go to it is all."

"What do you mean, Ralph?" Tom asked.

"Well, suicide is always an option," replied Ralph. "It is the ultimate expression of self-control and independence. Biblically sound. There's not one verse in the Bible – Old Testament or New – that condemns suicide. In fact, in the Old Testament Great King Saul is said to have committed suicide after losing a battle to the Philistines. In the early church, killing yourself was not considered a sin, and this law of personal freedom is clearly set out in the Greek Code of Justinian. St. Francis of Assisi prayed:

> *Our Sister Bodily Death,*
> *From whose embrace no living person can escape.*
> *Happy those she finds doing your most holy will.*
> *The second death can do no harm to them.*

"Did you know, Tom, that every year over a million humans on planet Earth commit suicide? That's twice the criminal murder rate. No one can say that killing yourself is not a very human response to life's disappointments."

"You're not thinking about harming yourself, are you Ralph?" Tom asked in a concerned voice.

"No, friend Tom – at least not yet," said Ralph. "The Romans may have surrounded Masada, but we're not yet ready to spoil their psychological victory. I've decided on another tact."

"Which is what?" asked Tom.

"Which is," answered Ralph, "to adopt the life of the Desert Fathers."

"Prayer and fasting?" asked Tom.

"No! Dear boy," exclaimed Ralph Simionedes. "I'm going to drop out. My sessions with the psychiatrist are over. Cooperation with the pharaoh-establishment is over. I will model myself after the famous monk Arsenius who fled the life of a wealthy aristocrat of the senatorial class in Rome to become a monk in the Egyptian desert. I've read about him. We all have. He made my trials and tribulations in this hospital seem ridiculous and picayune. He gave away a fortune to adopt a simple lifestyle in the desert. Then he inherited a second fortune, and when a legate from Rome brought him the news all the way into the desert, he refused the inheritance on grounds of his 'death' eleven years earlier. You see, he had long since committed a type of living suicide to the rules and regulations of the establishment. Arsenius was not necessarily depriving himself of sustenance or suffering and mortifying his flesh to get closer to God. Rather, he was effectively 'turning off the receiver' of hypocritical modern life in his own time so that he could hear God speak. Arsenius was well educated in both Greek and Latin and yet went from being an urbane and rich city dweller to making baskets and selling them for pennies for a living."

"How will you live in the desert in this place?" asked Tom.

"Friend Tom," replied Ralph, "no one has to transform this place into a desert. It *is* a veritable desert. We are many, many miles from a society that will accept us as *bona fide* citizens of it. In fact, such a society may not be in this life. I will commit myself to Helios in my desert called the Northwest Iowa State Hospital, but I reserve my right to commit myself to the eternal Helios in death. Life is not sacrosanct, friend Tom. Death is. A meaningful death is much more significant than a meaningless life. Dame Juliana of Norwich prayed to receive the sufferings of Christ *'unto death'* on her thirtieth birthday, and it was only through her experiences at the very threshold of death itself while in severe pain that she experienced the ecstasy of God. The Aztecs sacrificed living people to Helios – who they worshiped under the name Tonatiuh. The Druids sacrificed willing victims to Helios at Stonehenge at the first rays of the winter solstice."

"Death is the great equalizer, friend Tom," continued Ralph. "All humans fear non-existence, and they want to know that their ego-selves will, in some way, transcend their own deaths. If they *knew* this for certain, then maybe death would not be considered so hysterically bad after all. If religion of any variety was so thoroughly convincing that mankind was assured of its continued existence post-death, and of the fact the post-death continuance of existence would not be painful, then religion would serve at least a psychological benefit of calming the death-anxieties of humans. This would be helpful even if false religion were founded on pure fantasy and had no correlation with reality whatsoever. Then the argument of atheists like Dr. Feingold might be 'there is no God and no existence after death, but at least organized religion is doing a *good thing* by calming people's fears about death.' However, calming people's anxieties is *not* the intent of organized religion in the most popular beliefs in the world. These religions gain converts and keep organizational attendance by *creating* anxiety and then offering to take the anxiety created away through institutional religious attendance. The punishment for 'sin' (*i.e.*, transgressing God's law) is still 'death' as was the punishment for most lawbreakers in the Torah or Old Testament. But, in Christian and Islamic theology the 'death' prescribed is now *permanent in everlasting hell*. A sort of life-death. How little do these people understand the healing power of death. How little do these people understand Helios, forever radiating. Forever burning, and in death we return to the source of all power. But, friend Tom, you understand Helios, don't you?"

"Yes," replied Tom. "I understand. But, Ralph, if . . ."

"Shhhh," said Ralph interrupting with his right index finger pressed to his lips. "Silence. 'Strength is to sit still, sayeth the Lord.' Remember the Quaker prescription for the Inner Light: 'Be still and listen.' Then the Uncreated Light will come. Then you will know what to do."

Tom looked up to see that Ralph had left the room.

As he sat in the sunroom watching the moths circulate around the three lights of the billboard that evening, Tom determined that he would follow the path of Ralph Simionedes. It was useless trying to communicate with Dr. Feingold. Dr. Feingold would twist around everything he said. There was only one real and permanent way he would ever get to leave this horrid place. If only he were two hundred yards closer to the highway. But he would fast. He would pray. He would 'commune with his own heart' as the Bible said until the Uncreated Light came to him. Most of all, he would not fear the death that is to come, for in a way death was not death but freedom. A freedom of the ultimate sort and a uniting with Helios, the Uncreated Light of all creation.

Chapter Twenty-Four

Tom's symbolic retreat into the desert began rather slowly. For a time, he continued to drink coffee and smoke Newports with Maggie Mae in the wing's dayroom at one of the tables, and to discuss various things. For a time he even spoke to the nursing staff occasionally, although he never again spoke a word to Dr. Feingold after a particularly distressing session he had with the doctor one Monday in which the doctor had brought along with him an editorial which he had clipped from the Sunday *Madisonville News-Ledger*.

"I thought you might like to hear an editorial I spotted in the Sunday paper," the doctor had said. "It's entitled '*Woe to You Scribes and Pharisees, Hypocrites*.'"

"Want to hear it?" the doctor asked.

"It's your show," replied Tom. "If I say 'no' you'll tell the Judge I was 'uncooperative'."

Ignoring Tom's remark, the doctor began:

We have watched with interest, and frankly at times with encouragement, as an up and coming non-denominational group operating the Church in the Fields grew from a few members meeting in an old barn north of Madisonville in early 1986 to what is now a sizable church even by Des Moines standards with – we are told – over 3,000 registered members. But with the growth in Church attendance has come the predicable growth in monetary contributions to the various so-called 'ministries' of its leader the Reverend Kevin Dykes.

It has recently come to our attention that this same Reverend Kevin Dykes was reported in the St. Paul Democrat, our sister paper to the north, in its March 3, 1985 issue to have had a serious falling out with the elders of his previous congregation over the handling of church funds, and specifically concerning the purchase of several expensive items, including an electrically heated dog kennel and Jacuzzi for his home's back yard. Reportedly, a lawsuit was headed off by the production of documents by Reverend Dykes showing that he and his wife Mary Ann were the only actual members of Guidance Tabernacle Ministries, the organization which collected all contributions from the faithful and was the owner of record of all of the church property.

The loophole, or perhaps the foresight of Reverend Dykes, successfully averted a lawsuit, but made continued service in the vineyard of St. Paul, Minnesota, by the Reverend questionable.

Although investigative journalism is more the bailiwick of big newspapers like the New York Times and the Des Moines Leader, our interest was piqued so we called the Secretary of State's Office and sent someone to the courthouse to examine the deed of the fairly recently purchased property comprising the Church in the Fields sanctuary. Sure enough, the non-profit organization 'Church in the Fields Ministries' shows that one "Reverend Kevin Dykes" and "Mary Ann Dykes" as being the only actual members of the organization, the only members of the Board of Directors, and the only Officers. Of course, they are! They elected themselves. Their non-profit is the registered owner of the church building north of Madisonville. And sure enough, there are now the first rumblings of alleged misuse of church offerings and financial gifts to line the closets and driveway of the Reverend and Mrs. Dykes' home.

In answer to the allegation that Church funds have been used to purchase $2,000 tailor-made suits, and among other things a set of diamond cuff links for his French cuff shirts, Reverend Dykes is reported to have compared his wardrobe quite unfavorably to the priestly garments festooned with jewels which were commanded by the Lord for his priest Aaron to wear in the Book of Exodus. By comparison, we are to suppose, the Reverend Dykes is downright shabbily dressed! And then there is the $65,000 Winnebago Mr. and Mrs. Dykes propose that their non-profit purchase for them – complete with an oversized refrigerator so that Mrs. Dykes can transport her (and undoubtedly justified) famous potato salad along with her husband to 'the more remote areas of Iowa' to 'pastor small churches' as visiting clerics. The last time we checked, after the invention of the automobile, no place in the State of Iowa was in the slightest degree 'remote,' and as far as we are concerned no church in this State – regardless of size – needs the type of pastoral services specialized in by the Dykes.

> The philosopher Santayana is quoted as saying "Those who cannot learn from history are doomed to repeat it." Far be it from this newspaper to suggest where a citizen ought to worship his or her God. Our job is only to – and in only rare instances – point out what will be found when you get to a particular place.

Dr. Feingold put down the article and looked at Tom.

"What?" asked Tom. "What do you want me to say?"

"I don't want you to say anything," replied the doctor. "What I want you to possibly realize is that 'God' as you envision him or her does not necessarily move through Reverend Dyke or by means of this whole notion that the Old Testament Yahweh – this same Neolithic notion of a revengeful god who slaughters whole populations and commands his own followers to kill (in one instance an only son) – is possibly not the same God that ultimately inspires you to worship, engage in prayer, and perform activities such as that. Tom, no one is persecuting you for your beliefs – even to the point of hearing the voice of someone or some force you reckon to be God within your own mind or heart. What is totally *unacceptable* is the thought – or fear on the parts of those charged with your care and who are concerned about you – that such a voice could command you to harm others or yourself. Do you understand the distinction?"

"No," said Tom. "What you are suggesting is that a person – that is a sane person – ought to exercise *control* in some ways over how God will act or what God will tell you. If God exists as *an other*, separate and apart from individuals, how can that be? I can't control how you act or what you elect to tell me."

"The 'other' concept of God does not exist in all religions," replied the doctor. "For example in Vedic, Hindu and Buddhist traditions humans are thought to be a part of the ultimate whole of a good god – or reality – and so when it comes to moral choices and actions one is to act in a way consistent with beliefs that his or her god is essentially benevolent. It is nearly impossible for the believers in these traditions to believe that their god will throw themselves some kind of curve ball one day and say 'go act *malevolently* towards your neighbor. The time has come to kill him'."

"You want me to become a Buddhist?" asked Tom.

"*No, Tom!*" Replied the doctor. "I do not want you to become a Buddhist. I want to learn *discernment*. I want you to convince me that the God you know and listen to – the God who dictated your book to you . . ."

"The Uncreated Light," interrupted Tom.

"The Uncreated Light," the doctor agreed nodding his head, "is not such a God or entity or voice who would tell you to harm others or yourself, and if you heard such a suggestion – either out loud or within yourself – you would be highly skeptical that the voice was genuine, and it would not be genuine because your god is incapable of such a suggestion."

"Maybe if I was a Buddhist, I could do that, Doctor," said Tom, "but I am a Christian. The same type of Christian who listened to St. Augustine in the Fifth Century when he argued that God approves of a morally 'just war,' in connection with which the killing of others is no sin. I am the same type of Christian who heard from the priests in the Middle Ages that it was no sin to kill a Jew or an Irish human being. I am the same type of Christian who was given advance and total absolution for all of the Islamics I would kill in the crusades in order to win back the Holy Land for Christ."

"Well, you're certainly a clever Christian," said the doctor. "I'll give you that. And now you're going to ask me why the Northwest Iowa State Hospital is not filled to capacity with Christians who believe what they are told about their god, even to the extent of killing others?"

"In response to which you will reply," said Tom, "that most Christians don't claim to hear the voice of God – literally, that is. But isn't there hardly a Christian cleric alive – notwithstanding pentecostal prophets and prayer leaders by the tens of thousands – who doesn't claim God speaks to them, has spoken to them or – God forbid, Doctor – commands them through the literal pages of the Bible?"

"I don't know, Tom," said Dr. Feingold, "and I'm historically at a complete disadvantage discussing history with a historian, but State Law makes no exception for Christians or any other practitioners of various beliefs with regard to the criteria of admission in here. I have never held the opinion that the world religions – all of them in fact – were anything less than irrational and illusory. I just do, that's all. You have your beliefs, and I have mine. But, Tom you flunked the litmus test of schizophrenia and you won an admission ticket to this place as far as I was concerned when you audibly heard one or more voices that no one else can verify hearing and you admitted that you might – even might – act on the instructions of those voices to harm yourself or others. I'm not bound by the code of evidence the court in Madisonville as in a legal case. I don't care about legal precedent. I care about you, and in your book, you outright said the Holy Spirit or whatever . . ."

"The Uncreated Light," said Tom interrupting.

"You *said*, Tom," the doctor forcefully replied, "the Uncreated Light dictated the book to you, and then you told me you might very well have to do what the Uncreated Light told you to do – even under extreme circumstances. Do other Christians believe God talks to them in very plain and audible ways? I don't know. Maybe a great many of them do. I'm not sure I would run off to a holy war without some kind of motivation beyond a preacher's urging – but I'm not a Christian. I never was, and I'm quite sure I never will be. Maybe a great many other Christians would sacrifice their own children or kill others if the voice they believe is God's told them to. Other Christians are, so far, not my responsibility. You are."

"So, I got myself into this jam by being an honest Christian at the wrong place and at the wrong time," said Tom.

"You're not in a jam, Tom," replied the doctor. "You are in a State Hospital – and not a bad one as they go, by the way – because I believe to the best of my professional opinion that you are a threat to yourself or others. And you are not going to get out of here until I am convinced that you are at least beginning to doubt the reality and veracity of any voice that speaks to you privately and out of the hearing of others, especially if those voices suggest depressing or violent scenarios. Tom, it's no fun being a doctor and losing a patient to a whispering and suggestive voice – and it doesn't make things any easier if the patient thinks it is God's voice as opposed to the devil's or Hitler's or anything else."

"This is a waste," said Tom. "The integrity of my mind is all I have. You're not going to make me deny my own thoughts. I'm finished listening to you!"

Tom crossed his arms and turned away from the doctor. Not only this session, but all others with the doctor were ended as far as Tom was concerned. Words like "avolition" and "non-cooperation" began to be written into his chart, and on two occasions the word "catatonic" was noted. For a time, Tom ate, although always sparingly. Then for a time he ate less. And then for a time he ate even less. When the feeding tube was finally surgically implanted in his stomach, Tom never ate conventionally again.

During the mornings, Maggie Mae sat with him on the naugahyde furniture in the sunroom passing a pack of Newports back and forth. Then as Tom's condition worsened and the staff insisted Tom use a wheelchair to keep from falling, Maggie Mae would wheel Tom to the sunroom and put a Newport to his lips for him to puff.

Maybe it was as a consequence to the feeding tube being implanted – or maybe it was just Tom's imagination – but Ralph Simionedes began to show up for evening discussions less and less in the fall.

In the last week of October, Tom received a packet of mail from the University. It included the letter from Chancellor Post Tom knew would eventually come confirming his final discharge from the University, and also a sealed violet envelope addressed to *Tom Schmidt*, but otherwise without a return address or any other identifying mark. Inside, Tom found three lined and hand-written pages from Gloria Singleton. The letter read:

Dear Tom,

I am so sorry I took this long to write to you, but I had to find a way to communicate even if it is rather sneaky. I came to see you right after you were ~~tom~~ put into the hospital, but they wouldn't let me see you. They said that I was not on the "approved visitor" list that included "anyone from the Church in the Fields, and especially Reverend Dykes and Gloria Singleton." I don't know why they included me, but they did. They said the prohibition also included any written communication of any kind or phone calls. I tried writing once, but the letter came back in a large envelope from the hospital administration. At least they hadn't read the letter. Anyway, I am slipping this letter into the campus mail they are supposed to bring you, but without a return name or address. I hope it reaches you.

Tom, I want you to know we are praying for you – and not just me but the whole church – the prayer line, the small group prayer warriors, everyone. Pastor Dykes even gave a special sermon in your honor three Saturdays ago. He preached that you, more than anyone in Madisonville he knew of, had suffered reproach, ignominy and exclusion for the sake of Jesus Christ – and happy would be your reward in heaven, because they had treated the prophets the same way.

Pastor Dykes has suffered too – not only in being prohibited from coming to you and pastoring you himself – but because of the newspaper article and the lawsuit. I suppose you heard about all of that.

Anyway, we are doing <u>great</u> at church. We have purchased a large RV and painted all across both sides of it 'Holiness to The Lord' (Exodus 39:30). Each week a ministry team takes the RV with a load of potluck dishes and food, and they go around the State to encourage little congregations just getting started. One of the music ministers plays the guitar, and then either Elder Cecil or Elder Dave breaks open the Word and preaches. Then everyone enjoys the potluck. We take everything – plates, silverware – everything, and we clean it all up for the people we visit too. I went with the team two weeks ago – we go on Sundays – to the New Leviathan Church in Elk Grove. It was FABULOUS! I felt the Spirit of God course through my veins, and I thought I was so possessed by the Spirit that I would die! Anyway, it's been two weeks, and I'm still buzzing.

Before I forget – I saw your boys the other day at that McDonalds by the South Gate of the University. I'm sure it was them. They were in there with someone I didn't recognize (maybe a male relative?) Anyway Sueann (?) was not there with them. They are so cute! I do hope you get to see them regularly.

Get well! That's an order! Actually, and truly, the Lord Jesus has told me that "Tom Schmidt will suffer, but for every moment of suffering, he will be exalted a hundred-fold".

Tom, we all love you so much. Can you write? If you can, PLEASE write. If you have to, send letters to my next-door neighbor

Gladys Toler, 444 Europe Street, Madisonville 50125. She's not on "The List" and I've clued her in that she might be receiving a letter for me. Get well, Tom.
    Love, Gloria

Chapter Twenty-Five

Then, on one December afternoon, Tom's old acquaintance Sammy showed up with a Hispanic-looking sidekick named Carlos.

"Are you ready to see the Judge?" Sammy asked Tom somewhat in passing as he grabbed the handles to Tom's wheelchair, swung it around from Tom's vista of the stubble-strewn barren cornfields, and began pushing the chair down the hall.

"Judge?" asked Tom.

"Yeah, Judge," replied Sammy. "The same Judge we went to see in the spring. They thought they could have a hearing without you, but they beeped me and told me the Judge had thrown a fit and wanted you there."

"Oh, that Judge," replied Tom. "I guess it *has* been 180 days. I've lost track of the time."

"Where's Mick?" asked Tom as Carlos held back the elevator doors and Sammy pulled his wheelchair into the elevator.

"You mean Nick?" asked Sammy, and then without waiting for Tom's answer said, "Nick went to Chicago. He got a job at Cook County and supposedly he's doing real good. Got him a new pick-up truck and everything."

"Good for Nick," Tom said.

Unlike Tom's previous experience at the Madison County Courthouse, there was no waiting or isolation in store for him this time. Sammy and Carlos escorted him in the wheelchair up the courthouse elevator, down a short hall and through the grimy stained double doors of a very large – and for the most part empty – courtroom. At one of the tables up front sat the attorney Nora Minden, and next to her sat Dr. Feingold. Near the Judge's elevated bench, a man in uniform stood talking to a female court reporter sitting before one of the shorthand machines Tom recognized from re-runs of *Perry Mason* on television. However, the Judge was nowhere to be seen.

When Ms. Minden noticed the wheelchair and its entourage, she rose to her feet and said, "Mr. Bailiff, please go get the Judge. He said he wanted to be notified promptly when Mr. Schmidt arrived."

In about ten minutes there was a loud rapping on the door next to the Judge's bench, and the returning Bailiff called out formally, "all rise."

Judge Giddeon walked into the courtroom swiftly behind the Bailiff, but on the way to the bench the Judge stopped and began to stare at Tom in his wheelchair with the two attendants.

"Damn it!" Judge Giddeon exclaimed. "Gerry, come up here. Lisa, this is off the record including my inappropriate comment."

Dr. Feingold stood up and walked over to the Judge, who was still standing by the bench at the front of the courtroom.

"Judge, Judge, don't get upset," said Dr. Feingold in a loud whisper. "He's taken a turn for the worse."

"Turn for the worse?" said Judge Giddeon with an disgusted look on his face. "Gerry, against my better judgment I let you have this guy for a work-up. A work-up, Gerry. Now the Patient Advocate is calling the Chief Judge saying he wasn't given a copy of the Evaluation and Treatment Plan or even notified of this hearing, and Mr. Schmidt here looks like they just brought him from Auschwitz."

"Your Honor," said Nora Minden from her place at the table.

"Sit down, Ms. Minden!" the Judge called out, not looking up.

"Judge, he stopped eating," whispered Dr. Feingold. "We had to insert a feeding tube to keep him alive. You signed an Order for Involuntary Nourishment and Medication ten weeks ago."

"I signed an order?" asked Judge Giddeon.

"Yes, Judge," replied the doctor. "You signed it, and the request spelled out the guy's condition."

With an exasperated throw of both hands into the air, the Judge announced, "Mr. Bailiff call this case" as he climbed the three stairs into his seat at the bench, and Dr. Feingold walked back to the seat next to Ms. Minden.

"Oh Yea, Oh yea, Oh yea" said the Bailiff in a loud monotone voice, "in Case Number 89-0056, In the Matter of Thomas Alvin Schmidt, the court is back in session. Please be seated."

"Ms. Minden," said the Judge. "During the lunch recess did you call Mr. Clifton Lamonte like I asked you to?"

"Yes," replied Ms. Minden standing. "I was able to reach him, and I expressed the Court's concern that he was attorney of record for Mr. Schmidt and was not present at the 180-day hearing as scheduled this morning."

"And?" asked the Judge.

"Well, Your Honor," replied Ms. Minden, "Mr. Lamonte related to me that his clients were the Reverend Dykes and the Church in the Fields, and not Mr. Schmidt individually, and that he had received neither instructions nor a retainer fee for progressing further with the representation of Mr. Schmidt at this point in time."

"Is that right?" asked the Judge incredulously.

"Yes, that's right, Your Honor – almost verbatim," replied Ms. Minden.

"Well, Ms. Minden," said the Judge, "I just really don't know about that. Excuse me for my demeanor, Ms. Minden, but I – that is the Court – is extremely upset over these developments. In the record I have before me there is no signed return or waiver for this hearing from the Patient Advocate, and the Patient Advocate is not here. Maybe my seventy-three-year-old eyes are failing. Do you see the Patient Advocate here, Ms. Minden?"

"No, Your Honor," the woman replied.

"And I see in the record no motion to withdraw representation submitted from Mr. Lamonte relative to this case. Did he call you, Ms. Minden, and tell you he was formally withdrawing?"

"No, Your Honor," replied the woman.

"Perhaps the Clerk misplaced it – did he send you a motion and order to withdraw from this case?"

"No, Your Honor," replied Ms. Minden.

"Leroy," the Judge called to the Bailiff. "Go downstairs and send a squad car over to pick up Mr. Clifton Lamonte, Esquire, and put him in that holding cell down the hall. I'll be finished with my other business about 5:30 this afternoon, and then we'll see what we'll do with Mr. Clifton Lamonte, Esquire for failing to show up in court either this morning or this afternoon because he had no instructions from the Church in the Fields or its preacher. I think the Iowa State Bar Association may have a different understanding of an attorney's duty to his client than does Mr. Lamonte – but we'll see."

The Bailiff disappeared through the door at the rear of the courtroom.

"Now gentlemen," the Judge said, "be kind enough to wheel Mr. Schmidt down to me, and I'd like the record to reflect that Mr. Schmidt is wheelchair bound and is frankly emaciated in appearance since he was last in this courtroom."

"Judge!" Dr. Feingold exclaimed rising from his chair beside Nora Minden.

"Sit down, Dr. Feingold!" the Judge replied gruffly. "The court has a few questions for the psychiatrist in this case, but not just yet. Resume your seat, Sir."

Dr. Feingold sat down just as the Judge looked up suddenly and toward the back of the courtroom.

"What do you need, Deputy?" the Judge asked.

"Judge, I'm from the process section," the Deputy answered.

"You got somebody to serve with papers in this courtroom?" the Judge asked.

"Yes, Sir," the Deputy answered. "We found from the docket that Mr. Thomas Alvin Schmidt would be in court today. We've been holding process on him for three days because we can't serve him at the . . ."

"Yes, I know," said the Judge. "What kind of process is it?"

"A petition, Your Honor, for Divorce from Bed and Board," the Deputy said.

"Oh Lord," said the Judge. "Well here he is – get on with it."

The Deputy advanced to Tom's wheelchair and placed the papers into Tom's hand. "I'm sorry, Mr. Schmidt," the Deputy said quietly.

"You did your duty – skedaddle," said the Judge to the Deputy.

"Mr. Schmidt," said the Judge, "You're a hell of a sight, Sir. Lisa, keep that one on the record. What's happened to you in the last six months?"

Tom was silent.

"Mr. Schmidt, if you so desire, I can appoint an attorney at law to represent you in these proceedings. Is that your wish?"

Tom vaguely moved his head in a negative signal.

"What's this man's medication, Dr. Feingold?" the Judge asked.

"Haldol intra-muscular, Your Honor," said Dr. Feingold rising from his chair. "Bi-weekly with his last injection ten days ago."

"I want him off all medications for another ten days," the Judge said in a stern tone. "And I want him back in here, this Thursday a week at 9:30 a.m. I want you here with him, Dr. Feingold. Due process for zombies is not my specialty. If we're going to do something we might as well do it right. And Ms. Minden, I want you to type up this order yourself along with an order that the Clerk assign independent counsel at county expense for this man for the next hearing, and then walk it personally over to the Patient Advocate's Office. While you are at it, drop off a copy of the Evaluation and Treatment Plan submitted in this case. The patient Advocate claims he didn't get a copy. If the Court receives a request from the newly appointed counsel for a continuance of the hearing prior to twenty-four hours of its schedule, the Court will grant that continuance for two weeks without a hearing. I am issuing a second order – we will prepare this one Ms. Minden – that an attorney at law customarily practicing family law before this court be appointed at county expense to represent Mr. Schmidt here relative to the matter he was just served with. The court *ex proprio motu* is granting the to-be-appointed attorney forty-five days to respond to this suit during which time on motion of the defendant it will be determined if he is capable of cooperating with his own appointed counsel despite the previous orders of the court and/or whether he is sufficiently destitute financially to justify further representation at the county's expense. Since this man is under interdiction and State supervision, I am ordering that his family matter be transferred to my division for all further proceedings. Mrs. Thomas Alvin Schmidt is hereby prohibited from making any and all financial decisions on behalf of her husband or alienating any joint property, including sums of cash on deposit, that is not exclusively titled in her name. Make sure she is served with a copy of this order, pronto. That is all. Since we temporarily have lost our Bailiff, court is dismissed."

The Judge stood up and began to gather papers from his bench desk.

"Judge," said Dr. Feingold walking around the table at which he was seated.

"Court is dismissed, Dr. Feingold!" the Judge said gruffly, and he turned and walked out.

Chapter Twenty-Six

The next morning Tom awoke to find Maggie Mae sitting by his bed.

"Quick, Tom," she said. "I'm not supposed to be in a male patient's room. Let's get you into your wheelchair and go down to the sunroom."

At the sunroom, Maggie Mae reached into the pocket of Tom's hospital issue faded green robe and pulled out a half full packet of Newports.

Pulling two out cigarettes out of the pack, she lit hers and Tom's, and then put one of the cigarettes between Tom's lips, saying "Well baby, you made history around here. According to the spic who brought you up here you cleaned Feingold's plate in court yesterday. Zip! Zip!"

"No, I don't think so," said Tom exhaling through clenched teeth.

"Yes, baby. It's a good story – don't mess it up," said Maggie Mae.

"Are they really taking me off meds?" asked Tom between clenched teeth.

"I don't know, baby," replied Maggie Mae. "I thought you didn't take that stuff."

"They shove it down my tube and inject it. Instant psychotropics," said Tom smiling with the Newport still clutched in his teeth. "The bastards won't even let me die."

Tom laughed in between puffs and coughed between his still clenched teeth.

"Tom, baby, don't say that," said Maggie Mae taking the cigarette out of Tom's mouth and replacing it with a freshly lit Newport from between her lips. "You don't want to die like that poor bastard on the bridge."

"What poor bastard?" Tom asked.

"It's in the Sunday paper. I found it in the trashcan at the nurse's station and I took it to my room. I always like to read about the weddings."

"Go get it for me, would you Maggie honey?" asked Tom, tilting his head and with some effort taking the cigarette from his mouth with his left hand.

Within two – or three – minutes Maggie returned with several sections of the Sunday *Madisonville News-Ledger* folded in half in her hands.

"Let me read about the poor bastard," said Tom.

"Tom, I don't think . . ." said Maggie Mae.

"Give it to me, honey," Tom said shortly.

Tom read silently to himself:

> *Police have now discovered the identity of the man who hanged himself from the Little Otoe River Bridge south of Madisonville last Wednesday evening. He has been identified as Professor Ralph Simionedes of Davenport.*

"That's sad, isn't it baby?" Maggie Mae said. "All those kids and his farm. You're not going to try and hurt yourself like that clod-hopper now, are you Tom baby?" Maggie Mae asked as she threw her arms around Tom in his wheelchair. "They say – that is the bastards say – that a lot of us schizophrenics commit suicide. Tell me you're not going to hurt yourself Tom!"

Maggie Mae was hysterically beside herself as Tom stared straight ahead.

"No Tom, no Tom!" Maggie Mae screamed. "Don't hurt yourself."

Within a minute a large built nurse's aide appeared from the hall, put a strong arm around Maggie Mae, and said, "Mrs. Thurstan, Mrs. Thurstan – calm down!"

"I shouldn't have done it! I shouldn't have done it!" Maggie Mae screamed. "I thought it would help. I gave Tom the story about that hick on the bridge who committed suicide and asked Tom to never hurt himself, but I know Tom will try and hurt himself – I can see it in his eyes."

"Mrs. Thurstan," said the woman, "The man *fell* from the bridge. The man *fell* from the bridge. He didn't jump deliberately. Mr. Schmidt is starting twenty-four-hour watch on orders of Dr. Feingold this morning. Nothing's going to happen to Mr. Schmidt."

"Bitch!" screamed Maggie Mae. "What do you know?"

With all of the commotion a male orderly appeared and began to wheel Tom back down the hall towards his room.

"It's going to be O.K., Mrs. Thurstan," said the woman aide in a kindly voice, guiding Maggie Mae towards the nurse's station.

When Tom was pushed back to his room, he found on his bed yet another University Mail yellow envelope, inside of which was only one piece of mail. It was a letter from The Church in the Fields to "Associate Professor Tom Schmidt, Room 202 Allen Hall, Harvest Christian University, Madisonville, Iowa 50125." Tom wondered if the mail prohibition had been lifted or whether this letter had got through without being screened. Inside a larger white business envelope was a smaller self-addressed envelope to the attention of "The Church in the Fields," and a letter on Church stationery signed by "Rev. Kevin Dykes, D.Div." It read:

Dear Fellow Yokesmen,

As the season of Christmas draws near, it is most appropriate for all of us to take time to pause and reflect on the many blessings we have received throughout this past year. Father God is faithful and true. The Lord Jesus Christ answers prayer, and He has answered our many prayers and petitions without number this year. The Holy Ghost comforts us in our afflictions. Indeed, we have seen our congregation grow and prosper this year to an unprecedented extent. If everything works out, our Planning Committee tells me we can break ground on our new Sanctuary in the Fields on the first of March of this coming year.

But, Beloved (and truly each and every one of you is Beloved), our needs are great. There is much work to be done in God's harvest of souls — a fact that is constantly brought to mind for each of us as we worship in the midst of the seasonal changes in the corn fields all around us. Only recently we were required to replace the aging Oldsmobile of the Pastor's wife, and to the celebration of the heavenly host we have now purchased and have in operation our 'Prayer Mobile' that spreads news of the 'renewing of our minds' (Romans 12:1-2) to the farthest corners of the State. But also, the expenses mount. We are now paying our nursery ministers to provide childcare, *and we have experienced some legal fees and expenses.*

Although it is a pleasure, Beloved, to offer our tithes and offerings to the Lord, we need to remind ourselves frequently that it is also our **bounden duty** *to give unto the Lord to the full extent of our capacities to sacrifice. I am reminded of the Prophet Malachi's warning to each of us in Chapter 3, Verse 8 of his prophesy:* **'Will a man rob God? Yet ye have robbed me. But ye say, wherein have we robbed thee? In tithes and offerings.**' *Tithing is not enough! Holy scripture makes it quite clear that both tithes <u>and</u> offerings are necessary in order to avoid even the semblance of robbery in the eyes of the Most High.*

Therefore, if you have not **tithed** *the full amount to the Church this year, I admonish you as your Pastor concerned for your spiritual welfare to do so without delay. An envelope addressed to our Church is provided in this letter just for that purpose. If you have fully tithed this year, it is now time to prayerfully* **give offerings** *unto the Lord. In good conscious I cannot thank you for doing what the Lord God has commanded you to do. As Mary Ann and I prayed at our kitchen table together as man and wife for the strength to do what* **additionally** *was right for our Church this last week, and when the check was finally written and we had placed it into the same envelope as you are receiving, we both nodded our heads in agreement with the humble servant described in the Gospel of Luke (17:10), "When ye shall have done all those things* **which are commanded you**, *say 'we are unprofitable servants:* **we have done that which was our duty to do**'.*

God Bless You, and Merry Christmas,
The Reverend & Mrs. Kevin Dykes

When Tom finished the letter, he went over the table by his bed and, opening the drawer, reached far into the back for a small piece of tissue wrapped around twelve pills he had hidden there some weeks ago. He also retrieved his wallet and seventy-six cents in change he found in the corner of the drawer. Pulling the eight remaining dollars from the billfold, he placed the paper currency and the seventy-six cents in change into the envelope in the Church's packet. Turning his back and unwrapping the pills, he surreptitiously dropped the Haldol into the envelope.

"Can you get a couple of stamps for this?" he asked the aide sitting in the green chair now on the other side of the room.

"Sure, Mr. Tom," said the aide looking up from her *Women's Day* magazine. "I have some in my purse. I'll even mail it for you on my way home."

"Thanks," replied Tom.

That Sunday afternoon Father Ben Grey stopped in to see Tom in his room but finding him not in, he was about to leave when he noticed Tom at the end of the hall in the sunroom. The priest walked to the end of the hall and saw not only Tom in his wheelchair, but a tall blond orderly sitting in one of the chairs reading a copy of *Sports Illustrated*.

"Patrick, could I have a minute or two with Mr. Schmidt alone?" asked the priest.

"Sure," said the young man. "If they ask for me, I will be laying out toiletries and a new bathrobe for Mr. Schmidt on his bed."

"Tom, how are you doing?" asked the priest laying a hand on Tom's shoulder.

"I guess O.K.," said Tom. "Do you mind if I smoke?"

"No," said Father Grey. "I don't mind if you smoke. Can I help you?"

"Yeah, said Tom. "The Newports are in the pocket of my robe. It's kind of twisted around. They take the belts off the robes they deliver to E-Echo and it's hard to keep everything in place."

"Yes, I know," said the priest reaching into the robe's pocket between Tom's wheelchair and his thigh.

The priest took the flattened pack of cigarettes and a pack of matches from Tom's robe pocket, put a cigarette into Tom's mouth, and struck a match.

They say," said the priest putting the match to the end of Tom's cigarette, "that you are in a very bad way."

"What do *they* say, Father?" asked Tom. "*They* don't tell me much around here."

"Well *they* say, Tom, that you might be having kidney problems. *They* say you are definitely having problems related to not eating. *They* also say that you are suicidal. Tom, *they* don't say – but I say – that my dear friend Tom Schmidt may be very near death. That's why I'm here, Tom. My friend Tom Schmidt seems to be dying – and despite everything I know and everything I believe and every word of the Christian faith I cling to, I don't think I have helped him."

"Thank you, Father," said Tom through clinched teeth holding the cigarette. "Is there something like last rites in the Episcopal Church?"

"There is," said the priest.

"Will you read them to me?" asked Tom.

"If you insist," replied the priest opening his small black leather prayer book, "but I'm not sure it is in order."

Reaching his hand over to Tom, the priest placed his finger tips on Tom's forehead and said, "Almighty God, look on this your servant, lying in great weakness, and comfort him with the promise of life everlasting, given in the resurrection of your son Jesus Christ our Lord. Amen."

"Amen," said Tom. "That's it?"

"Under the circumstances, Tom," said the priest, "that's it."

"Father, I've thought a lot about abortion and death and things like that over the years," said Tom. "I know that Job had the strength of a saint – but is it possible that God could just give a man the nod? I mean, I've lost everything, and I don't know why. My job. My wife. My boys. My sanity. Even my self-respect. Do I have to take this forever?"

"Life is to live, not just to endure, Tom," said the priest. "All I can tell you is that one of the many writers of the Bible – a man who was searching for a meaning to life just as you search – wrote: "to him that is joined to all the living there is hope, for the living know they shall die, but the dead know not anything."

"God bless you, Tom," said the priest, rising. "Patrick is coming back now. I see him down the hall."

"Father?" Tom asked.

"Yes?" said the priest.

"What does that billboard say across the road?"

"The billboard?" asked the priest.

"Yeah, the billboard," said Tom. "You know it's getting to the point where I can't always trust what I see and hear."

"Well, Tom, it says," replied the priest, "Hayes County corn growers can count on super yields using Easy Spray 38 – 1. I suppose that is some kind of fertilizer or chemical."

"38-1?" asked Tom turning his head to look himself.

"Yes, Easy Spray 38-1, Tom," said Father Grey.

"I was hoping it didn't say that," replied Tom, "but I see you're right. Easy Spray 38-1."

"Is there some significance to that, Tom?" asked the priest as the orderly arrived.

"No, not really," said Tom. "It's just a sign."

Father Grey walked slowly beside Tom's wheelchair as the orderly Patrick pushed Tom down the hall toward his room. When the group had nearly arrived at Tom's room, Father Grey suddenly stopped and placed his hand on one of Patrick's hands grasping wheelchair grips.

"Patrick, stop a minute please," he said. "Just stop right here."

Kneeling down in front of the wheel chair, the priest reached out and made the sign of the cross on Tom's forehead, and said, "deliver your servant, Oh Lord Christ, from all evil, and set him free from every bond, that he may eternally rest with all of your saints in their diverse eternal habitations where with the Father and the Holy Spirit you reign, one God for ever and ever."

"Thank you, Father," said Tom.

With tears in his eyes, the priest rose, and patted Tom's hand on the armrest of the wheelchair. Nodding, he turned and walked toward the nurse's station.

After pushing Tom's wheelchair into his room, Patrick maneuvered it over to the bed.

"Goody, clean everything and a new robe no less," said Tom looking at the items on his bed.

"Do you want me to put them away?" asked Patrick.

"No, I'm not helpless," answered Tom. "They just don't like me to leave the room without the wheelchair. I'll put everything away."

"Oh, Patrick," called Tom a moment later. "I'm all out of Newports. Be a good lad and go up to North Echo 112 and bum a pack from my friend Maggie Mae."

"That's Alice Thurston's room," replied Patrick.

"No, I'm sure you'll find Maggie there," said Tom.

"Mr. Schmidt, I'm not supposed to leave eye contact," said the orderly.

"Patrick," said Tom in a pleading tone of voice. "I've just been with a priest confessing all my sins. I need a smoke, for Christ's sake. Please just run upstairs and bring me a pack. Tell Maggie I love her."

As the young man was walking out the door to the room, Tom called, "Patrick, please close the door – I'm going to put on the clean pajamas."

Tom pulled the big door shut.

Getting up from his wheelchair, Tom pulled off his robe and pajamas and threw them in a pile next to the wardrobe on his side of the room. He opened the door to the wardrobe, and with a scoop of one arm pushed all of the clothes hangers on the cross bar to one side. After dressing in the clean pajamas and new robe he walked over to his bedside table and picked up the styrofoam pitcher, pouring water first over one hand and then – exchanging pouring hands – over the other.

Kneeling down in front of the open wardrobe, he held up both his hands in front of him, and said, "Lord?"

"I'm here, Tom," a voice answered.

"I did everything you said," replied Tom.

"Well done, good and faithful servant," said the voice.

"May I now, Lord?" Tom asked with tears running down his cheeks.

"Yes, Tom," answered the voice, "You may now enter into my eternal rest."

"Thank you, Lord," said Tom dropping his hands to his side.

Almost miraculously, the fingers of his left hand felt the dangling cloth belt of his new green hospital robe.